Method **P**utkisto

Marja Putkisto was born and brought up in Finland, and trained there as a fitness and dance teacher. It was while working at the Sibelius University of Music and the Finnish National Opera that she began to investigate muscle balance and movement in general. This led her to question the tightness and shortness of muscles in the human body. She began to study valuable techniques such as Pilates, and she worked in collaboration with Finnish sports doctors, physiotherapists and chiropractors. From this broad basis of knowledge, she developed Method Putkisto, a deep-stretching technique which is now used to improve the performance of sports people and performers, especially dancers, actors and singers. She came to London in 1990 to develop the use of the Method in the UK, and teaches it privately and in open classes. She is married, and lives in central London.

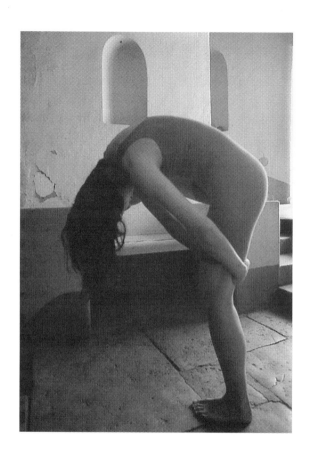

Method **P**utkisto

DEEP STRETCH YOUR WAY TO
A FIRMER, LEANER BODY

Marja Putkisto

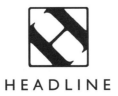

HEADLINE

First published in 1997
by HEADLINE BOOK PUBLISHING

10 9 8 7 6 5 4 3 2 1

ISBN 0 7472 7760 5

Typeset by Clive Dorman & Co.

Printed and bound in Great Britain by Mackays of Chatham PLC, Chatham, Kent

HEADLINE BOOK PUBLISHING
A division of Hodder Headline PLC
338 Euston Road
London NW1 3BH

CONTENTS

DEDICATION

To my father, Professor Kalle Putkisto, who taught me the value of curiosity.

ACKNOWLEDGEMENTS

Book Photography

Principal Photographer: Kari Hakli

Art Director: Marja Putkisto

Set Design: Anu Hakli

Make-up: Sirpa Lipponen, Sari Happo, TainaWetterstrand, Soili Kuhanen

Hair: Marco/Point, Helsinki

Clothing: Piruetti, Reebok

Venues: Finnish National Opera; Finnish Castle, Helsinki; Inkoo Islands,Finland; Hersham residence, London

Models: Ulla Mannila, Yumi Iwasa, Petri Toivanen and Jarkko Niininen (Finnish National Ballet), Jari Tuomola, Heidi Mattila, Heini Putkisto, Kare Hyvärinen, Eva Virta, Hanna Virta

Assisting Models: Pirkko Jalava, Heikki Lempiäinen, Juha Karvonen, Olli Pietila, Aida Hersham, Marja Putkisto, Maria Gripenberg, Matti Vilppola, Kumi Ishihara, Jane Mulholland

Additional Photography (pages 2, 9 and 47): Kaj Ewart/Studico

Drawings

Yumi Iwasa

Writers

Tisha Harrington (main text), Gillian Mosley, Hans Svenheim

Editor

Susan Fleming

Book design

Clive Dorman

Book cover

Photographs: Kari Hakli, Stephen Benson

Make-up: Lynn Rae

Design: Jon Morgan

Logo design

Jarmo Lehtonen

A BRIEF BIBLIOGRAPHY

Kehon Rakenne, Toiminta ja Lihashuolto, Jarmo Ahonen, Tiina Lahtinen, Marita Sanstrom, Giuliano Pogliani, Rolf Wirhed (Valmennuskolmio Oy)

Sana'ki, Terveydellinen Maailmankuva (Panasana Oy)

Anatomy, Henry Gray (Churchill Livingstone)

Atlas of Human Anatomy, Frank H. Netter (CIBA-GEIGY Corporation, USA)

The Thinking Body: Study of the Balancing Forces of Dynamic Man, Mabel E. Todd (Dance Horizons, New York)

Body Movement : Coping with the Environment, I.Bartenieff and D. Lewis (Gordon & Breach)

The Anatomy Coloring Book (Harper & Row)

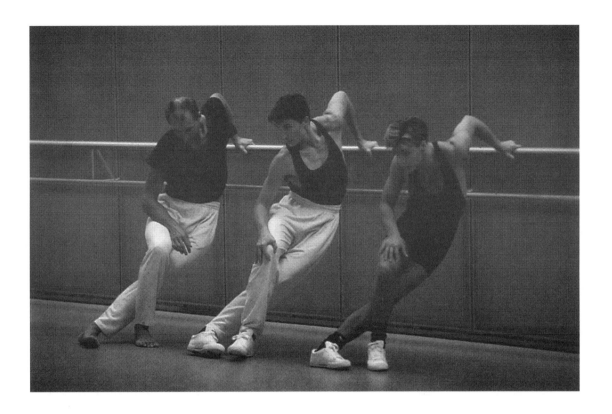

A NOTE

The exercises in this book are intended for healthy people who want to improve their level of fitness. However, exercise in inappropriate circumstances can be harmful, and sometimes even fit and healthy people can injure themselves. If you have any questions concerning your own state of health, consult a physician or other qualified health professional before following the instructions in this book. The publishers, the author and the photographer cannot accept any responsibility for any injury or damage incurred as a result of using this book.

I should also like to give special thanks to the following people who have been particularly supportive or who have influenced my thoughts during the process of creating the concept of Method Putkisto.

Yumi Iwasa	Anushka Boome
Hans Svenheim	Hanna Jones
Kari ja Anu Hakli	Anna Karvonen
Philippa Dickenson	Lucas Howing
Heidi Mattila	Carol Coff
Gillian Mosley	Gordon Thompson
Sally Tottenbier	Helena ja Taisto Oinonen
John Finta	Maria Gripenberg
Mette Heinz	Eila Tervahartiala
Jarmo Lehtonen	Lisa Spiro
Jari Tuomola	Keijo Kupiainen
Ulla Mannila	Päivi Ylänen
Jarkko Niininen	Ritva Löfberg
Inkeri Simola-Isaksson	Shazia Quraishi
Merja Makinen-Martindale	Jacqueline Korn, David
Kyllikki Lyytikainen	Higham Associates
Aki Loikkanen	Richard Gallafent
Eeva Kaario	Francis Mitchell

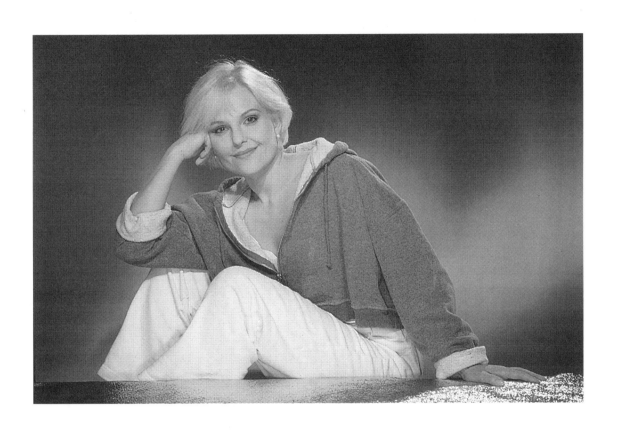

INTRODUCTION

'Small things together cater to perfection.
Perfection is not a small thing any more.'

MICHELANGELO

I grew up with a deep love for dance and music. Despite having been born with a hip displacement I was, even at a young age, searching for outlets for rhythms and movements which would flow freely with me.

For the first eight months of my life my lower body was held in a static position with my legs forced into a constant 90-degree position. After that my hip sockets were considered to sit properly. The problem was solved. I was thought of as a healthy, normal little girl. While I have no memories of early infancy, I was both physically and psychologically affected, and in fact the problem had only been solved at a superficial level. I grew up feeling confined, with a strong desire to move.

I lived in Finland, on an island in front of the open sea. In this part of the world, each of nature's constant changes of seasons is extreme – from the dark, long winters to the white summer nights. As I grew, I unavoidably developed an internal rhythm in synchronicity with nature that fed my desires and ideas for movement and music. Although I went on to pursue a conventional career in business, I remained drawn to the world of art until I came to terms with my inner drive to make it my profession in one way or other. I then began my studies in physical education and was introduced to voice training.

It was during one voice workshop that I was first struck by the notion of muscle imbalance. The instructor gave us breathing exercises that focussed on the lower back area. There I was, sitting with my hands around my waistline, and realising that breathing into my lower back was an impossibility. My awareness of my lower back existed only as a blind spot. I continued to carry this new realisation beyond the workshop until I began to make a curious connection between this and my struggles as a child to develop certain physical skills. As though watching a film, I began to remember the difficulties I had learning to throw a ball, swim, ride a bicycle etc. According to one teacher I was considered an ungifted mover. I also remembered the day when one of my ballet teachers explained I would never achieve the splits due to the way I was built. Needless to say, I was repeatedly disappointed with my progress. As a child I simply couldn't understand why some of the set targets seemed to be so impossible to achieve when I had such a desire to try.

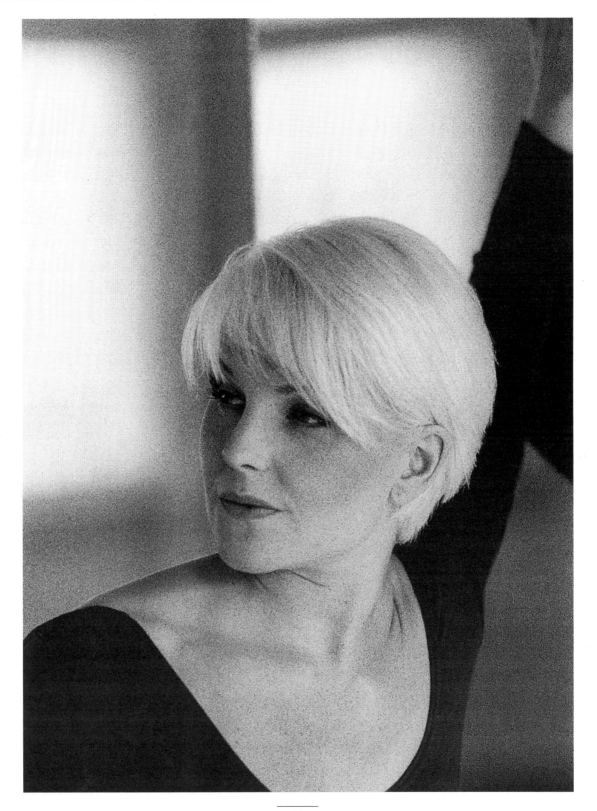

In search of answers to my questions concerning the blind spots in my body, I was able to find skilful teachers who noticed that the misalignment of my hip was still deep rooted. I had grown up and developed, with my body off centre. Due to the feeling that one side of my body was too short on the inside, I started searching for knowledgeable doctors, physiotherapists and osteopaths who were able to further my vocabulary and create a more concrete picture of what had previously been only an abstract concept. Based on the knowledge I gathered at this point I knew that the only way to overcome my imbalance would be to literally stretch my shortened muscles into the length which would finally allow my hip to move freely. That was the beginning of the Method Putkisto deep-stretching programme, and my motivation to study the human body and its motor skills in depth during the following years.

Method Putkisto places an emphasis on opening and lengthening muscles which are too tight and short, unlike conventional exercise which can result in *shortening* the muscles. This enables you to achieve suppleness, strength, balance, well-being and awareness. In order to get in touch with your body, you must understand the basic muscle mechanisms (see page 21). This makes it easy to stretch them or strengthen them. Through the developing stages of Method Putkisto, I realised that the most effective way of overcoming the defence mechanisms of the body (see page 22) was through following a sequence: visualising the chosen muscle and then, in a stretched position, allowing the body weight to deepen the stretch with the flow of the breathing. Understanding this concept removed much of the mystery of my own body. It became more concrete, yet malleable. The question of the out-of-shape body became answerable since I was able to reshape my own body completely. This process of taking responsibility for my physical situation gave me great independence and understanding of the physical setback which had hindered my overall development.

At 26 years of age I began working at the Finnish Opera House and Sibelius University of Music as a movement and dance specialist. Here I had the opportunity to work in an environment where the performers worked to reach a level as close to perfection as possible. Noticing that some of the movements and postures of the performers were restricted, I started working on my ideas regarding the question of tight and short muscles in relation to opera singing as well as ballet and dance. During the following ten years of working with a dedicated group of people, the visible changes were so significant I realised I had taken the right direction. Method Putkisto proved itself able to help maximise the body's capacity to improve quality of movement and voice. My work acquired a new seriousness.

So far the programme has been used to improve the muscular coordination of people like dancers, singers, musicians, parachutists, polo players, football players, runners and hurdlers. It has also been successfully used by individuals of all ages to increase fitness levels and overcome aesthetic body problems by reshaping waistline, legs, buttocks, chest, breasts and face. It is helpful for overall well-being by improving digestion, breathing capacity and circulation, and decreasing cellulite. I now feel a never-ending amazement and respect for the human body's capacities to heal and correct itself, when it is given the opportunity to do so.

This manual outlines *fifteen steps* to which you apply the *five elements* of a deeper stretch. Each step highlights different muscle groups or emphasises another aspect of the movements associated with stretching. At the beginning, you will find a selection of suggested stretching *menus* to use as a guideline for your personal programme. These menus are only to serve as a framework, or starting point for structuring your own programme from the material presented in the steps. You should never feel that you are solely limited to the material I present.

You will also find that incorporating deep stretching into your overall fitness programme enables you to reach measurable improvements in your progress. I want to emphasise that you need a balance between cardiovascular (aerobic), strengthening and stretching exercise. However, out of all the components which contribute to your overall fitness, flexibility is the quickest to gain and the easiest to maintain. It can be the missing link to accessing your physical targets and aesthetic ideal.

METHOD PUTKISTO

Its Principles, Your Awareness

METHOD PUTKISTO STATEMENT

Flexibility is the link to your body's strength and balance. In principle, each muscle should be longer than the bone whose movement it initiates or supports.

Muscles tend to stay in shortened positions because we sit for hours a day, year after year. These shortened muscles eventually force the body out of alignment. This can lead to problems like ribs slowly sinking towards the pelvis which leads to loss of waistline, loss of abdominal support, shoulders rolling forward and the head sitting in an incorrect position. To correct misalignment, Method Putkisto offers you the following programme which reaches beyond the 'normal' stretch to a deep stretch. Method Putkisto is based on the use of *focus, time* and *weight,* creating the dynamics for the stretches that actually *lengthen* your muscles. Increased flexibility improves the well-being of your body, 'lifts' you to a better posture, and facilitates freedom of movement. Through Method Putkisto deep-stretching exercises, you can redesign your body to reach its aesthetic ideal.

YOUR AWARENESS

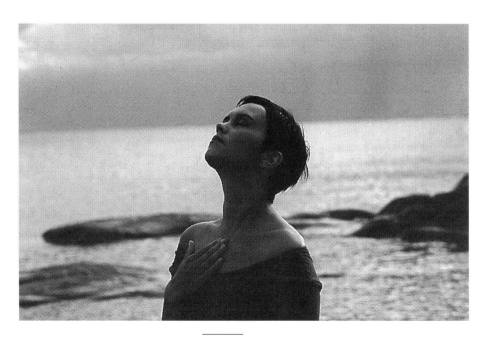

Your inner awareness of your body is the product of a chain of various experiences that you use as conscious or unconscious guidelines in different situations. It is attainable at many levels and in many areas of your life. You can expand it throughout your life, but you can also lose touch with it, depending on your choice of lifestyle. Building body awareness is an ongoing process which relates to being in touch with your physical age, your weaknesses and strengths, your gender and sexuality. It also relates to aspects like your spatial awareness (how you move through space), your use of body weight, and how you use such awareness in different situations and in relation to different people. How aware are *you* of your body?

* Do you have a realistic and healthy image of your body?
* Do you have control over the fitness level of your body?
* Do you know what your physical weaknesses/strengths are and why?
* Are you aware of your current physical state in respect to your age, and are you setting your targets too low or too high?
* Do you know how the different muscles in your body work together?
* What part of your body do you use to initiate your various movements?
* Do you follow certain movement patterns?
* Do you have the vocabulary to make decisions and choices for your body, or do you rely solely on the opinion of other experts?
* Are you aware of your physical needs, i.e. when you are tired, hungry, etc.?
* Do you have the knowledge to guide the pace of your body, either to speed it up or calm it down?
* For women, are you aware of and in accord with the cyclical changes in your body, i.e. monthly, pregnancy, menopause, etc.?

If you have sufficient vocabulary and understanding of your body, you are capable of making decisions that are relevant to your body. In a physical sense, you can achieve results and progress in much less time. You don't simply exist in your body, you control it. Then as various elements take effect – for example force of gravity, different cycles, time – you begin to understand them, respect them, connect to them, and use them to your benefit.

If you lack this awareness you can be very vulnerable when adjusting to changes in your body. You are more likely to make inefficient decisions, and the results of your physical targets can be poor. Your body will remain a mystery to you.

As you progress through the Method Putkisto deep-stretching programme, you will gain an awareness of your body in relation to stretching. To help you to master this, I have included the following terminology and concepts for you to study. Many of these appear throughout the book. Those that do not are still important to keep in mind. You may periodically refer back to them to improve your stretch technique while you work on your body.

TERMINOLOGY

MIND
Your mental existence; awareness; consciousness and unconsciousness.

Body Image
The visual picture of how you define your body in your mind; your perception of your body.

Focus
To focus is a conscious action to draw your attention, for instance, on, from or towards something. Your focus may alternate from the inside to the outside or from larger to smaller. Deep stretching requires you to focus your attention on the chosen part of your body.

BODY
Your physical existence and instrument.

Torso
The body excluding arms and legs.

Spine
The line of 24 vertebrae in the centre of the back, starting at eye level in the skull, running vertically through the ribs, through the waistline and pelvis, ending at the tailbone. Your central nervous system runs inside the spine through its core.

Tailbone
Coccyx; vertebra at the lower end of your spine.

Sitting Bones
The bones you sit on; the ischium; lower pelvic bone structure; origin of the hamstring muscles.

Pelvic Floor

Muscle layer between tailbone, sitting bones and the pubic bone. It initiates and secures the flow of all movement from the tailbone, particularly in the forward stride.

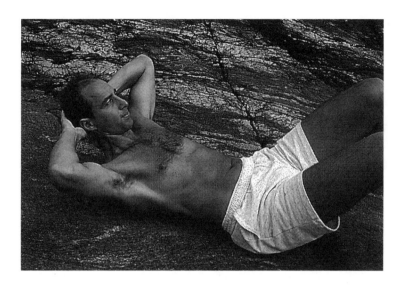

Abdominal Corset

The muscular support for your waistline; the space between your lowest rib and pelvis. It is the same area you engage when doing a proper sit-up. Refer to Half-Moon Breathing and the Warm-Up section, no. 3, for instructions on how to locate and strengthen your abdominal corset.

Hip Flexors

These muscles connect your legs to the pelvis and spine. When you contract them, they will flex your hips. These muscles tend to dominate the abdominal corset when doing sit-ups if the pelvis is not in a neutral position.

Note: Maintaining a centreline position keeps the pelvis neutral. It is tilted neither forward nor back. Refer to the definition of Centreline.

Lungs

The lungs are located inside your ribcage above the diaphragm. They begin underneath your collarbone and continue down towards your lower ribs. To focus clearly during breathing it is helpful to divide them into *the upper part of the lungs* and *the lower part of the lungs*, until you master the breathing techniques.

CONCEPTS

These will help you to focus and learn how to use your body while working through the Method Putkisto exercises.

Centrepoint or Solar Plexus

The inner area located four finger spaces below the bottom of your breastbone.

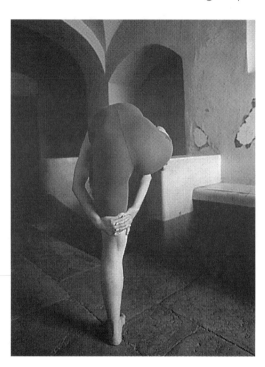

Centreline

This refers to the body's relation to gravity. The centreline runs down from the top of your head passing through your solar plexus and pelvis to the ground.

Ground Point

Point where you use your physical weight to harness gravity. This must be defined in relation to each individual or particular stretch. The ground point is used to help you increase, control and stabilise your stretches, and creates the opposition of movement that maximises them.

Back of the Ribs

The awareness of this area comes from lying on your back and allowing your weight to sink toward the back of the ribcage (the same as the base of your ribs). Practice of the concept helps you to become more in touch with the idea of being able to relax the muscles towards your bone structure.

Back of the Pelvis

Sacrum; awareness of this place comes from lying on your back and allowing your weight to sink towards your pelvic bone.

TECHNIQUE

Engaging the correct dynamic (use of time, weight, space; see Dynamics below) and focus for achieving a particular style of movement or performance. The more developed your technique is, the more power and control you can generate with ease.

Breathing

Inhalation of oxygen, exhalation of carbon dioxide. Breathing techniques are crucial in Method Putkisto.

Delay

DELAY is a pause or hold at the end of an inhalation or exhalation which creates a 'rolling into' the next breath. This aids in maximising each stage of stretching.

Stretching

Increasing the length of a muscle. Stretches are created through the use of dynamics.

DYNAMICS

Your body's use of time, space, flow and weight creates the dynamic qualities in your movement. Control over dynamics enables you to create a deep stretch.

Time

Quality of movement ranging along the continuum from slow/sustained to quick/sudden. Time spent in a stretch can be varied to achieve a set target.

Space

There is space inside and outside your body, as well as above and below, and to the side, front and back of it. This includes the dimensions: width, height, depth, and whether on the horizontal or diagonal. Movement can travel in space in direct or flexible lines. A sense and understanding of space is crucial for stretches.

Flow

Movement quality ranging from bound and controlled to free flow. Attention to flow is needed while stretching, so there can be a sense of ongoingness and change. The flow of your stretch follows your breathing (see Breathing, page 24).

Weight

This refers to the mass of the body which tends toward the centre of the earth because of gravity. Movement involves transferring your weight. Control and use of your body weight creates movement qualities along the continuum from strong to light and active to passive. Passive use of weight creates heaviness.

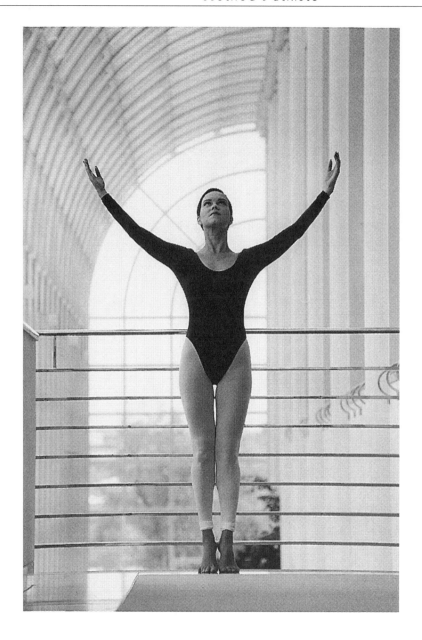

Space

ACTION

Stretching is an action (see Technique), as is holding still, doing something, transferring weight, falling, extending, contracting, jumping, tilting, looking up, looking down, etc.

Dropping of Weight

Getting in touch with gravity to sense your body weight and utilising it for either stretching or defining movements. Leaving the muscles passive to allow a sense of heaviness.

20

Strengthening

Making muscles stronger by working against force or weight.

Opening

Moving two bones apart, taking two or more muscle endings further away from each other; lengthening; the feeling of widening or spreading in relation to the space around you and within your body. (See Opposition of Movement, page 23.)

Centring

The conscious act of connecting to your centreline, using your inner spatial awareness in relation to gravity. You can do this either passively, through imagery or movement, or actively, engaging your postural muscles and abdominal corset.

Tilting the Pelvis/Initiating from the Tailbone

Use of the tailbone as an initiation point to curve, tilt or rotate the pelvis either up towards the navel or down away from it (see Flat-Back Pelvis Tilt on page 42).

ADDITIONAL STRETCHING CONCEPTS

The following include more specific stretching concepts that either connect or disconnect you from your stretching effort.

Muscle Mechanisms

The only action muscles can perform is contraction. They work in *oppositional pairs*: when you contract one group of muscles, the opposite group will relax. For instance, if you lift your forearm from the elbow, the muscles at the front of your upper arm – the biceps – are contracting, while the muscles on the back of the upper arm – the triceps – are relaxing. This is *involuntary* (see page 26), and to understand this is the crux of any stretching.

Muscle Memory

The muscle 'memory' of your body is the result of a lifetime of experience. It is the range and types of movement your muscles have developed based on your experiences and which are stored in your brain. The dimensions of the vocabulary you learn can be your choice. Repetitive movements do not encourage increasing articulation of movement patterns. You can train your body using ranges of movement to achieve progressively more defined articulation for each muscle group until it is implemented into your muscle 'memory', i.e. learned to the point where it becomes automatic, existing in your brain. Keep in mind that range of movement can be restricted by defence mechanisms and physical capabilities.

Defence Mechanisms

Overall resistance towards a new unknown, both in physical and mental terms. Your body's defences against being placed into unfamiliar positions are sensations of pain and biting points. To reach a deep stretch, you must overcome the inhibiting contraction which leads to a biting point and pain. Use breathing to relax your muscles. Once your muscles are relaxed the biting point will be overcome and the pain will fade, leaving you with a slightly numb feeling. This is the time to apply additional weight that allows you to stretch the muscle to its new length until it reaches the next level of contraction.

Biting Point

A muscle's reflex to an unfamiliar position is to contract instantly. This physical defence mechanism is particularly strong in the shoulder and hip area. When muscles have been in a shortened position for a long period of time, the muscle 'memory' does not immediately allow for elongation. While this contraction, the 'biting point', is not necessarily painful, stretching can become more painful until the muscle relaxes.

Pain

Pain is your body's defence mechanism and is there to protect you. In Method Putkisto the pain which is referred to is merely the discomfort associated with stretching. It is recommended that you become positively familiar with stretch pain or discomfort, and learn to release it.

Good Pain

This pain is tolerable and constructive, and is overcome by breathing and consciously relaxing through the muscle in your mind until the pain subsides into a comfortable sensation. Deep stretching involves leaning and relaxing towards the pain level, to go beyond it, until it gradually disappears, and allows you to deepen your stretch. (See also Safety, page 35.)

Bad Pain

This is sharp, intolerable and destructive pain experienced if you have stretched beyond your tolerance level. It is important, however, to differentiate between good pain and bad pain tolerance levels. Stop at your *good* pain level.

Blind Spot

A part of your body you cannot make a connection with. In order to connect yourself, use the process of visualisation to pinpoint precisely the muscle you are looking for while stretching. Blind spots are important discoveries. Keep working towards them until you are able to feel these parts of your body. Only by making efficient connections will you be able to utilise them fully. (Often they are in the lower back and between the shoulderblades.)

Opposition of Movement

This involves moving sets of bones and muscle endings in opposite directions from each other, either actively or passively. Knowing the muscle mechanisms, you can actively contract one set of muscles to create space between two bones, moving them further away from each other. Alternatively you can passively apply body weight through an isolated muscle group without engaging surrounding muscles to create the same effect. Refer to the Active Stretch and Passive Stretch definitions for further explanation.

DIFFERENT WAYS OF STRETCHING

There are several different ways of stretching: stretch, deep stretch, active stretch and passive stretch.

Stretch

In a normal stretch the muscle will reach its *original* length. This takes about 30 seconds.

Deep Stretch

A deep stretch begins where a normal stretch ends. It takes the muscle to a new length by working at a deeper level and with different timing and dynamics. You work on the stretch for a minimum of 2-3 minutes, and up to 5 minutes.

Active Stretch

Achieved with technique by contracting and releasing the isolated muscle being stretched (the stretch is created at the moment of release), or by leaving the isolated muscle passive while surrounding muscles are used to create the stretch. Bouncing is not a form of active stretching. *With Method Putkisto technique you can carry this to the level of a deep stretch* (see The Five Elements of a Deeper Stretch on page 24).

Passive Stretch

Keeping the muscle passive while the stretch is created by an outside force, i.e. your own body weight, or that of another person. *With Method Putkisto technique you can also carry this to the level of a deep stretch* (see Pressure Touch, Partnerwork, on page 155).

THE FIVE ELEMENTS OF A DEEPER STRETCH

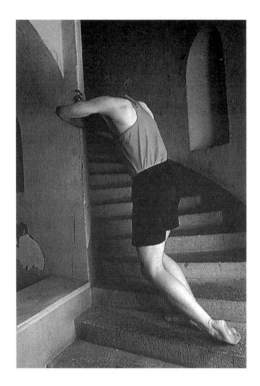

The principal elements required to create the correct dynamics for a deep stretch are *focus, breathing, space, weight* and *time*. By focussing on and isolating one muscle group at a time, Method Putkisto involves a combined use of time, your breathing and your own body weight to reach a deeper level of stretch.

I. FOCUS

Focus on a single muscle or group of muscles that you wish to change, one at a time. Set your target by visualising in your mind where the relative bones and muscles connect together. Imagine the muscle or muscle group lengthening and opening, and keep your centreline clear. Consciously relax the chosen muscle or muscle group. Work from the inside out.

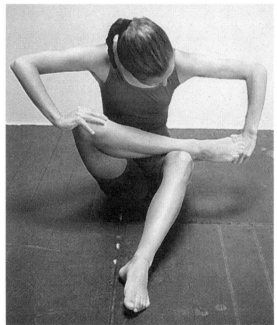

2. BREATHING

Your breathing creates the *rhythmic flow* for timing your stretches and contributes to the *pressure* of your stretches between breathing in and out. It also serves to *release* the discomfort of the stretch.

Focus your breathing into the isolated muscle. Feel the muscle or muscle group expanding from the pressure created by your inhalation. Exhale and feel the change of the pressure on your muscles.

3. SPACE

You create your stretch by moving your body in relation to the surrounding space. The stretches require awareness of the space around you. While working through them you need to know which part of your body is moving up and which part of your body is moving down to meet your ground point, which part is moving in towards your centreline, and which part is moving away from it (opposition of movement). Three-dimensional awareness provides a foundation that enables you to reach your targets (see Setting Up Your Own Targets, page 37).

4. WEIGHT

To create the stretch for the muscle to reach its new length you must apply sufficient weight on to it. You can use either your own body weight or an outside (partner's) weight. *The muscle or muscle group you have chosen to stretch must remain passive.*

By allowing gravity to take over, you can sink into a deeper stretch. By establishing your ground point, you can increase, stabilise or control the amount of weight needed for your stretches. You should aim to develop an awareness of your body in terms of sensing when and how much weight to apply. The isolated muscle will resist the applied weight (Defence Mechanisms, Biting Point, see page 22), but will gradually give in so that you can stretch it to its new length.

5. TIME

Take time to gradually deepen your stretch. No stretch will work unless your muscles are given time to respond to your conscious message to relax. Once your muscle has reached beyond the biting point to a more passive state, slowly stretch your muscle to its new length until it reaches its next stage of contraction or biting point. To reach a deeper stretch, the time required is longer than in normal stretching. Method Putkisto recommends that you work on the stretch for a minimum of 2 minutes, and up to 5 minutes. Avoid imposing a set time for the deeper level of stretch. Rely on your awareness. Listen to your muscle's responses, which will determine the timing.

WHAT YOU ACHIEVE

GOOD POSTURE

Posture is not a static state. It is a result of the dynamic relationship between our bones and muscles, voluntary and involuntary, which balance the body in relation to gravity. Discovering the links and connections in your body is an ongoing process. Your understanding and awareness of your body will expand as you make these discoveries and learn to respect the small inner components that can create this balance.

Bones

Bones provide the structural foundation for the body and its movement (your muscles are there to support and move the bones). Correct positioning of key structures like the pelvis is fundamental to complete body alignment. The pelvis acts as a base for the spine and as a bridge connecting your upper and lower body. When properly aligned, the legs sit comfortably in the hip sockets, distributing your upper body weight between two legs. Your legs are your connection to the ground.

Since your pelvis functions as a base for your spine, its tilt reflects the placement of the ribcage, upper back and shoulderblades. It is also possible to analyse visually the alignment of your upper body by using your collarbone as a measure. Your collarbone must sit horizontally in order for your ribcage, shoulderblades, and head to sit properly. If the collarbones sit in any angle of a 'V' shape, your posture is not properly aligned. The greater the degree of the 'V' angle, the higher up are your shoulderblades and the more misaligned your posture. The effects of misalignment are loss of waistline and of shoulderline as your shoulders roll forward. This causes the shoulderblades to move up, and your head to move too far forward or sink between your shoulders.

Once your muscles position your bones at optimum angles in relation to each other, gravity will act on them directly and your posture no longer requires muscular effort to maintain it.

Muscles

There are two types of muscles: voluntary and involuntary. The involuntarily controlled include the heart and arteries, lungs and intestines. The voluntarily controlled are the skeletal muscles, which are what we focus on in Method Putkisto.

Muscles serve to support and move the bones, protect the inner organs and keep us warm. Muscles should in principle be longer than the bones they move. If they are shorter, they will force the body into restricted positions. While the surface muscles serve primarily as protectors, it is the deeper muscles which maintain a lift in the body and articulation in movement.

The primary postural muscles are the deep hip flexors, the hamstrings and the pelvic rotators (the deeper buttock muscles). They connect the torso via the pelvis to the legs. The strength and length of these muscles in relation to each other contributes to the positioning of the pelvis and thus alignment of the body. The diaphragm also acts as a base for postural support.

The upper body is supported primarily by the big back, chest and abdominal muscles. Upper back mobility enables you to make the connection to the muscles between your shoulderblades: these open the chest and thus lift your posture. This allows you to make a connection between the latissimus muscles (see Note) and the abdominal muscles, which together create the abdominal corset around your waistline. Although a well-developed and maintained waistline exemplifies overall muscular balance, strength and control, it is crucial to get in touch with the deeper muscle layers as they provide a lift for your body and will prevent your weight from sinking into your legs.

Note: The latissimus muscles are the large back muscles beginning under the armpit and travelling down to the lower back.

FREEDOM OVER MOVEMENT

The efficiency level of your movement is reflected in just how long and strong your muscles are.

When one muscle becomes shortened, it remains short if its counter muscle is not used to its full range. For example, tight pectoral muscles on the chest pull the shoulders forward, thereby decreasing the ability of the chest to expand and limiting movement of the muscles in the upper back. Neither muscle group is working efficiently.

A good sense of your *pelvis* area gives you the foundation for achieving a higher sense of balance and quality of movement of your body. Your two *legs* operate independently from this single unit. The level of articulation of their movement is determined by the deeper buttock muscles and your hip flexors and extensors. If these are properly lengthened, they can lead you to a higher level of three-dimensional movement of your legs. Change in movement range is attainable by anyone, but the degree is dependent on whether you intend to exercise these muscles for everyday movement or for more complex purposes.

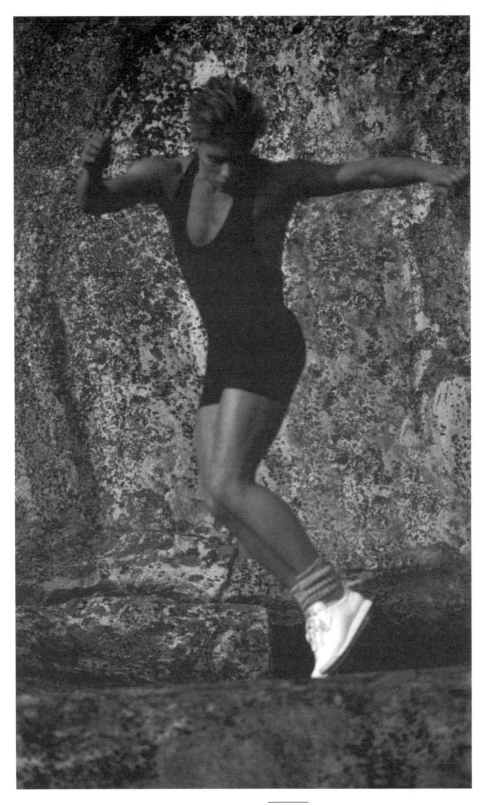

The flexibility of your *spine* provides the possibility for movement which requires use of your centre in all dimensions, i.e. curving, bending, reaching, etc. The spine runs upwards from your pelvis. It connects to your ribs, creates your neck and then connects to your skull.

The *chest* area, including your ribcage and shoulders, is related to the mobility of your *neck* and *head*. The chest must be open enough to allow the shoulders to fall back thus freeing the full range of movement in the neck. A misaligned neck and head affects your overall ability to develop proper techniques related to any sport.

Proper placement of the *shoulders and shoulderblades* affects movement of your neck and head as well as your arms. Efficiency and strength of arm movements rely on the connection of joints between shoulderblades and hand. If this connection is not defined, a weak muscular state develops and the arms will hang like a separate component from the torso.

Your muscles can either move you or inhibit your movements.

WELL-BEING

Posture affects your overall well-being. It also controls your ability to achieve the maximum level of fitness. When your posture is out of line, the use of the diaphragm is inefficient. Without efficient use of this primary breathing muscle, your body's breathing capacity will remain limited. This in turn affects circulation and metabolism. Your circulatory and digestive systems will slow down, which affects your body's ability to burn fat. Consequently, fat will be much more likely to accumulate on a body whose metabolism is not operating at full capacity. Moreover, if circulation through your body is limited, particularly to your neck and head, constant fatigue may result.

By using stretching to align your torso, you allow the respiratory and circulatory systems of your body to operate more efficiently and thus you will substantially *increase your energy level.*

Although it is not within the scope of this book to discuss which illnesses might occur from obstructed function of inner organs, we want you to note that there is such a connection between posture and health.

AESTHETICS

Individual aesthetics may vary according to your body image, your era, your culture and your upbringing. Whatever the aesthetics of your time, proper posture is the key to achieving the visual aesthetics regarding your physicality. If your alignment declines, this is likely to impair several of your body's physiological functions gradually.

When the ribcage sinks down towards the pelvis, there will eventually be a loss of waistline definition, as the postural support is missing. Shortened hamstrings will pull the buttock line down, and push the stomach out. The resultant shift in weight transferred from the torso and into the legs also begins to affect the shape of the legs from the thighs to the calves and ankles. Excess fat may then easily begin to accumulate as a result of ineffective circulation which is connected to poor diaphragm breathing. This connection to circulation affects even skin colour.

An open chest is a strong statement of your presence. The pectoral muscles cover the front of the chest. If these muscles become short they force your shoulders to turn inward. This will, in time, reflect the ageing process, as the naturally upright structure gradually becomes more stooped. If the pectoral muscles are lengthened they lift the chest and breast. Opening the chest limits underarm flab as well, by creating support for the arms by centring the shoulderblades on the ribcage and extending the shoulderline.

The chest is also a base for your neck and face. One of the problems that can result from tightness in the neck is the double chin. Generally a double chin problem is addressed with creams, facelifts, etc; rarely is the actual physiological aspect addressed. To eliminate a double chin there must be enough space between your chin and breastbone and enough space between the chin and the top of your throat.

There are three very common misconceptions about body shape, which are addressed by Method Putkisto. The first misconception is that tight, contracted muscles are strong. The goal should be the development of toned and elastic muscles, which are both supple and strong. The second is that the way to improve the abdominals is by scrunching them as we exercise rather than making a connection between the abdominals and deeper hip flexors, and then learning how to maintain control of these muscles while working toward a flat stomach. The third is that the buttocks can be reshaped and lifted by exercising the surface instead of the deeper layer of muscles (see Posture, Muscles).

You influence the physical aesthetics of your body through your physical use or misuse of your body.

HOW TO USE METHOD PUTKISTO

QUESTIONS TO ASK YOURSELF FIRST

1. What changes would you like to see in your body, in both appearance and performance?

For instance, would you like to lengthen your waistline, slim your thighs, shape your calves and ankles, widen your shoulders, align your ribs and pelvis, increase the flexibility of your back, hamstrings, etc.? Do you want to improve your sports performance (whether running, jumping or swimming), the use of your voice, or release tension etc.?

2. What is your body type? Soft and flexible or tight?

If your joints are overly mobile, your muscles may still be too tight and short. If you are of this muscle/body type, you will need to make more of an effort to focus on the

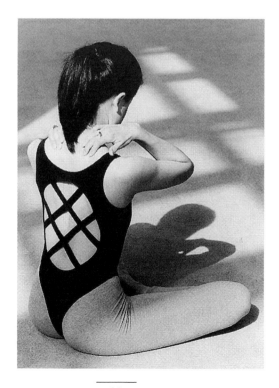

muscle group you are working instead of placing too much weight on the joints. Whereas if your muscles and joints are tight it might be difficult to get your body positioned correctly or comfortably before the stretch.

3. Are you aware of your habit of breathing?

Do you use the full capacity of your breathing? Are you using your diaphragm when you breathe? Do you tend to hold your breath in certain circumstances?

4. Are you aware of the location and amount of tension you carry in your muscles, and how this is affecting you?

Everyone carries some tension in their muscles. In fact, a certain amount is necessary; this is called muscle tone. However, too much tension is being carried if your muscles remain constantly contracted – for example, if your upper back muscles continually hold your shoulderblades too high. Over time, the lack of use changes the structure of the muscle, forcing the ligaments closer together and the muscle hardens to the point of becoming hard as stone. This type of muscle eventually becomes weak and fragile.

If you have this type of problem area, it might be effective to combine massage with your stretching programme.

5. What is your physical history?

Since early childhood, what has been your experience with physical activities? Have you had a physically active or passive childhood? Have these experiences been positive or negative? All of these have built the foundation for your current motor skills as well as your capabilities to learn new motor skills.

What injuries have you had? For each injury, there are two considerations: whether you have developed any protective mechanisms due to pain and muscle shortness, and whether there is any inhibiting scar tissue due to trauma or surgery. Because of the impact of a trauma it is possible to develop an unconscious protectiveness towards the injured part of your body. Over time, this constant mechanism influences your overall alignment. For instance, continuing to protect your shoulder beyond its injury will probably later lead to serious misalignment of the upper back and ribcage. Any time you incur even the smallest injury the healing mechanisms in your body produce protective tightness or scar tissue around the injured area. Any build-up of these can limit your mobility. One efficient way to change the negative effects following an injury is through stretching in order to increase mobility.

Note: In case of injury, apply the ICE principle. This implies Ice, Compression and Elevation of the injured area. As soon as this is done it will efficiently reduce the inflammation processes following a trauma, and facilitate healing of the injured tissue.

Note: Do not stretch a part of your body that is inflamed. Wait until the inflammation has been reduced. However, each injury and its procedures towards rehabilitation should be considered individually.

6. What is the present condition of your body?

What is your experience of physical training? Do you understand your body's signals and responses to training procedures? Have you reached a level of fitness you have been aiming for, or have you reached a plateau?

Have you noticed a gradual decline in your circulation?

7. Are you pregnant?

If so, be careful to stretch the hip flexor area, and keep the rest of your stretching programme at a maintenance level. Pregnancy can be a time when you are forced out of your centreline. After your pregnancy, the muscles around the pelvic area will remain soft and pliable for a couple of months. Use this opportunity to stabilise your lower back and maintain your waistline by working on the deep muscles that protect your spine and pelvis (see Posture, Muscles). These comprise the deep flexors and extensors and rotators of your hip joints. Obviously it is very important to strengthen muscles, especially those of the pelvic floor, after the pregnancy.

8. What is the muscle/fat/cellulite ratio of your body?

Select various parts of your body and gently lift the skin away from the muscle. Everything under the lifted skin and muscle is subcutaneous fat or cellulite. This will help you define your muscle and fat ratio. In areas where there is a concentrated level of cellulite and/or a reduction of muscle tissue, your circulation and, hence, your metabolism, is probably not functioning efficiently.

The problems of excess fatty tissue such as cellulite can be solved only from within by increasing your body's own metabolism. Cellulite accumulates easily in local areas like hips and thighs due to the short muscles and, thus, decreased circulation. In order to correct this, and hence the overall fat-burning mechanism, you must:

* increase the amount of blood circulation to that area of the body by stretching the short muscles.

* work on your breathing; e.g. aerobic exercises will increase your fat-burning mechanism to help build your body shape.

* maintain a balanced diet which will provide you with proper nutrition for your body.

9. What is your nutritional status?

The ability to strengthen and lengthen your muscles can be influenced by the quality of your diet. Healthy muscles should be mobile, and the tissue covering them, including the fascia, should be smooth and elastic. The signs of an imbalance in nutrition can be recognised as you stretch by pain – not 'bad' pain, but an uncomfortable type of pain that prevents muscles from relaxing into stretches. Other signs of poor nutrition include aching muscles and joints, dry skin, fatigue or morning stiffness.

To help your stretching you could consider the following nutritional supplements to begin with, particularly those which are highlighted.

*Vitamin B complex	– in particular, B12 for neural tissue
Vitamin C	– important for tissue renewal; anti-oxidant
Oils high in Vitamins A, D, E	– use of fish, sunflower, and olive oils will improve overall metabolic functions
*Magnesium	– to facilitate muscular functions like muscle contraction; nerve conduction
*Zinc	– necessary for cell growth and protein synthesis; increases enzymes in the stomach; strengthens tissues
*Silica	– improves the quality of the connective tissues in your body; preferably in gel or powder form

You may also be interested in adding the following supplements:

Amino acids	– elements in the proteins; important for rebuilding muscles; preferably in powder form
Enzymes	– break down food to increase absorption of nutritional agents
Lecithin	– breaks down fat molecules for use as energy source

Aloe vera drink	– includes lots of enzymes; strengthens immune system; detoxifies
Cider vinegar	– affects pH level of the body; diuretic; good for joints; detoxifies

Remember also to keep your sugar, full fat and white bread intake down. Drink lots of water. If you are unable to note changes or would like to know more about your nutritional needs, you can study specific information on diet or consult a nutritionist.

THINGS TO KEEP IN MIND

SAFETY

There is no danger in stretching if you work using the correct technique and the correct positioning of your body: proceed slowly and listen to your body (see Pain, page 22, and below). Allow your body to adjust to its new muscle balance in a relaxed position after the session. Stay warm. This makes your stretching safe.

Do not stretch inflamed or injured muscles. (See notes in above section on physical history for information on injuries and inflammation.)

After a deep-stretching session, you might experience a muscle soreness similar to that felt after an ordinary workout class. This is due to the muscles adjusting to a new length. As is commonly known, this is sometimes at its peak 48 hours after the workout. You can ease it by increasing your circulation, for instance, by gently stretching.

THE SETTING FOR YOUR STRETCH

The environment and space around you affect you more than you may know. Try various settings and see how you feel. Find one where you feel relaxed and comfortable, and which will help you to concentrate during your stretch sessions. You may want an airy space with plenty of natural light. You will need surfaces that provide support for your stretches (i.e. chairs, stairs etc). Wear comfortable clothing, and place something soft under your knees and back.

MALE/FEMALE BODIES

Muscle quality between the genders differs slightly. Men generally have more muscle mass while women have more fat tissue around their muscles. This implies that men must apply far more body weight on to a muscle in order to reach a deep stretch.

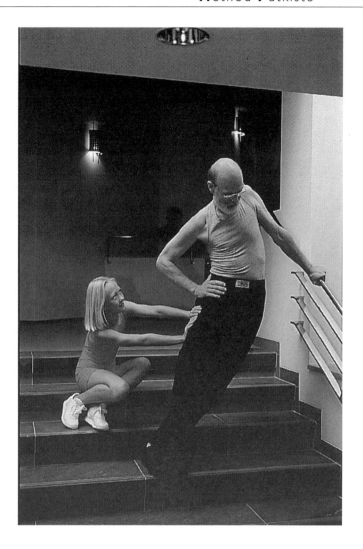

A G E

Whatever your age, do not under- or over-estimate your physical abilities or capacity to change your body. Your body continues to regenerate itself throughout your life. You can improve your level of fitness at any age. Set realistic targets for yourself.

O T H E R   E X E R C I S I N G

You will benefit most from your deep-stretching session if you combine it with light exercise or do it on a rest day, and then allow your muscles to adjust to their new length by resting. After a heavy workout, keep your stretches light. If you are competing, use deep stretching in the off season to improve your muscle balance.

MUSCLE BALANCING

Our bodies are not symmetrical on both sides: they differ in shape, size and placement, and they also differ in muscle shortness. As you stretch and become more aware of the varying degrees of shortness in your body, you will want to stretch the shorter muscles more intensively. For example, if you find that those on the right side of your chest are shorter than on the left, you could stretch the right side for a longer period of time than the left. *However, in general, it is important to work both sides equally.*

SETTING UP YOUR OWN TARGETS

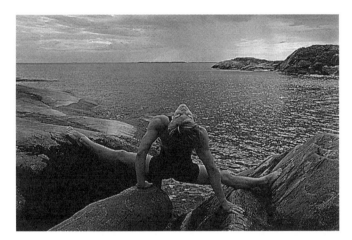

The following steps help you to set up your own targets.

1. Know Your Target

What do you want to accomplish with a stretch programme? Do you want to change your body shape, improve a certain type of movement, create a relaxation programme for yourself, achieve awareness or improve your well-being?

2. Choose Your Stretches

For each of your primary areas of concentration, select a suitable stretch related to your target. You might want to modify some of the ones presented in this book, keeping in mind the basic method of deep stretching.

3. Positioning

Although the position of each of the stretching exercises has been described for you in detail, keep in mind that by slightly shifting your body weight in the stretch position, you can create a different stretch. At a later stage, as your awareness and knowledge of your body increases, you can keep on exploring these possibilities.

4. Choose Your Frequency and Length of Time

Timing is crucial. Keep on working on each of your stretches for from 2 up to 5 minutes, depending on how deep a level of stretch you want to achieve. Repeat each of the stretches once a day for at least two months to achieve permanent results. Depending on the physical state of your body, you may be able to achieve permanency of muscle length with less frequent stretching, i.e. three times per week is commonly known as the minimum training needed for improvement of muscle length as well as overall fitness.

5. Evaluate Your Results

With the correct use of Method Putkisto, you will have *instant results.* You will feel lifted, open and relaxed. If the targets of the stretches you choose are clear, you should be able to evaluate your progress visibly after each deep-stretching exercise. For example, after stretching your waistline or hip flexors on one side, you will be able to see that that side is higher than the other when you stand up. If you cannot see any difference, the deep stretch has not been achieved.

In the long term, you will be able permanently to change the areas you have targeted. *Measuring the resting length* of your muscles indicates the *permanent results,* i.e. your muscle length when you wake up, before any exercise.

6. Maintenance

Once you have reached your target you have done most of the work. Maintain your new muscle length by using a normal stretch on the area one or two times a week, depending on how much you use the muscles. Remember, although maintenance is easier work than the process of reaching your target, the programme will remain successful only if it is used with the stated frequency. You can combine it easily into your normal fitness programme.

HOW TO STRUCTURE YOUR SESSIONS

Once you have established your target, based on your priorities, you can structure your own personal stretch sessions. As your awareness increases, you will develop a higher degree of sensitivity to your current state of fitness or flexibility. This awareness will lead you to re-evaluate your programme when necessary.

'MENU' SUGGESTIONS FOR STRETCHING SESSIONS

Note: For a shorter session, follow the programme marked with asterisks.

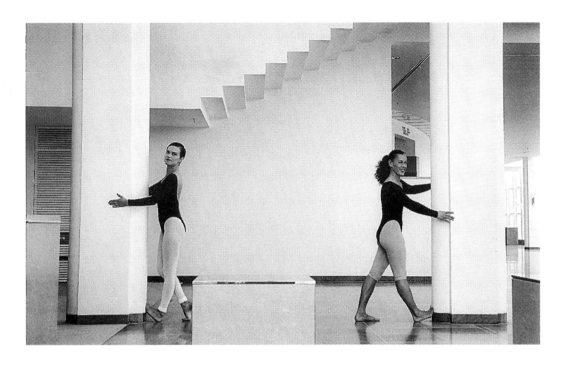

BEGINNERS		
1.	* Chest	L-Shape Press
2.	* Pelvis	Basic Lunge
3.	Pelvis/Buttocks	Sitting Lunge
4.	* Legs/Calves	Full-Body Tilt
5.	Legs/Back of Thighs	L-Pull
6.	* Neck	Long-Neck Stretch
7.	Neck	Side-to-Side Neck/Face Stretch
8.	Neck	Jaw Stretch

INTERMEDIATE

1.	*	Pelvis	Basic Lunge
2.		Legs/Front of Thighs	Rotation Lunge, Angles 1 and 2
3.	*	Chest	L-Shape Press
4.		Waistline/Abdominals	Bow Stretch
5.		Pelvis/Buttocks	Sitting Lunge/Standing Lunge
6.	*	Legs/Back of Thighs	L-Pull
7.		Legs/Calves	Full-Body Tilt/V-Tilt
8.	*	Back	Staircase Stretch
9.	*	Neck	Long-Neck Stretch

ADVANCED

1.	*	Pelvis	Basic Lunge
2.		Legs/Front of Thighs	Rotation Lunge, Angles 1-3
3.		Legs/Inner Thighs	Standing V
4.		Waistline/Abdominals	Bow Stretch
5.		Upper Back	Staircase Stretch
6.		Lower Back	Leg-over-Head Stretch
7.	*	Chest Stretch	Diagonal Press
8.		Arms/Biceps	Biceps Stretch
9.	*	Legs/Back of Thighs	L-Pull
10.	*	Legs/Inner Thighs	Standing V/Sitting V
11.		Legs/Calves	Full-Body Tilt/V-Tilt
12.		Neck	Cross-Arm Neck Stretch
13.		Neck/Face	Side-to-Side Neck/Face Stretch
14.		Neck	Jaw Stretch

EXPERIMENTS

Following are several experimental exercises which will help you understand the physical sensations and positions you will experience with Method Putkisto exercises.

NERVE STRETCH

The nerve stretch experiment is designed to give you an *awareness of your nerves* and the 'good' type of stretching pain that must be worked through. Your nerves originate in your brain and travel via your spine, branching out like a tree through your body.

Position

Stand or sit straight. Drop your head to the left, keeping your neck upright. With your elbow bent, flex your right hand, including your fingers. Begin to push the heel of your right hand away from the body to straighten the arm out to the side. Continue flexing the fingers backward, until you feel pain throughout the arm and towards the neck. You are now feeling the nerves and the kind of 'biting' sensation they will produce when you begin each new stretch.

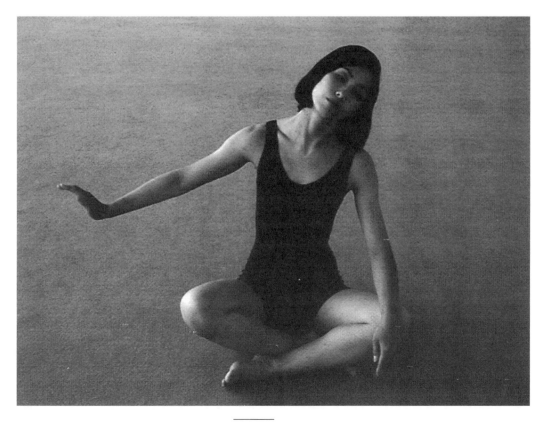

THE FLAT-BACK PELVIC TILT

This experiment is designed to maximise the various stretches. *Choose the degree of flat-back pelvic tilt related to the chosen stretch,* although in this experiment we will go all the way down to a horizontal position with the torso. Use your pelvis and torso as a single component. It is important to find the pivot between the pelvis and the hip joint as you tilt your tailbone away from your navel with a flat back. This helps you to isolate your legs from your torso.

Position

Standing upright, bend your knees slightly and begin to squat. As you tilt your tailbone away from your navel you are pivoting your pelvis from your hip joint. Maintain the length in your waistline and keep your back straight until your torso is horizontal. You may place your hands on your knees for support.

Note: If your weight is properly placed in your hip sockets you can extend your arms to your sides and still maintain your position.

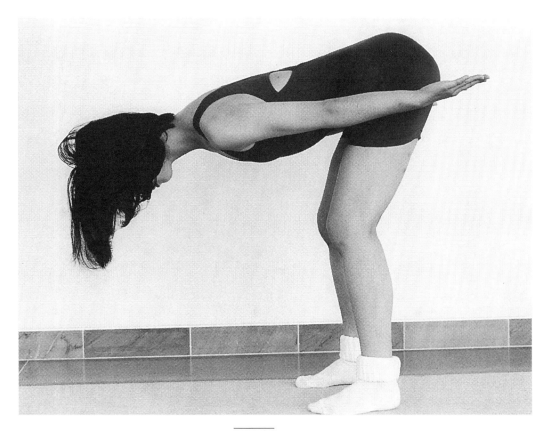

PRACTICAL APPLICATIONS

* Find the proper position to enable you to apply your body weight in a focussed way on to the muscle you are stretching.

* Identify and visualise the muscle you want to lengthen.

* Remember to keep the muscle or muscle group you are stretching passive.

* Use the appropriate deep-breathing technique to help open up the muscle or muscle group.

* Focus; send a message to the muscle to release it – at least 10-30 seconds is needed for the muscle to respond to the message to relax in order to begin your stretch.

* Take your time, and slowly stretch the muscle to its *new* length until you reach the next biting point. Decide if you want to deepen the stretch from this level.

* Listen to your intuition while you work through the stretches.

* Keep your movements small and precise.

* After stretching, stay warm and avoid exercise or other sudden movements; your body needs time to adjust to the new muscle balance.

THE FIFTEEN STEPS OF METHOD PUTKISTO

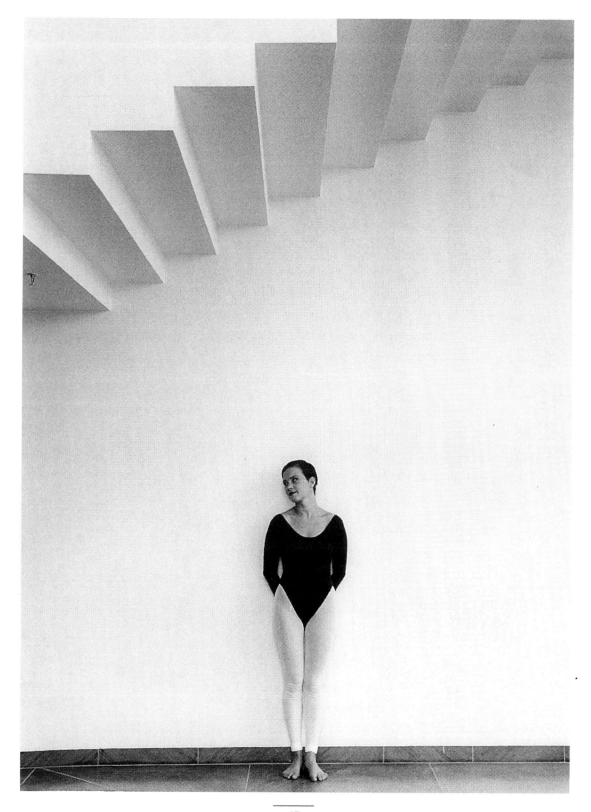

1

BREATHING

Breathing is your key to energy, vitality and power: you breathe to live. The inbreath or inhalation brings oxygen to the blood, and thus into the body to maintain metabolism and energy production. The outbreath or exhalation cleanses the body of carbon dioxide. Hence, one should aim to empty the deepest parts of the lungs where waste gas tends to remain. The body's postural support also becomes more readily available through efficient use of the breath.

In Method Putkisto, movement is initiated according to the rhythm of breathing. Breathing is the way to centre yourself and to focus on the area you want to work. In order to use the breath efficiently, it is important to know what the breathing muscles are, and to understand their action and movement. Different muscles are used for breathing in and breathing out.

1. The primary inhalation muscle is the diaphragm (inside the ribcage).

2. Assisting inhalation muscles include:

> – Intercostal (between the ribs)
> – Sternocleidomastoid (neck)
> – Levatore costarum (along the spine)
> – Scaleni (neck and shoulder)

Other inhalation muscles are in your neck, shoulder, between the scapulas (shoulderblades)and in the back and lower back.

Exhalation muscles include:

   – Intercostal (between the ribs)
   – Rectus abdominis (abdominal muscles)
   – Internal/external obliques (abdominal muscles)
   – Transversus abdominis (deep abdominal muscles)

Although different movement systems use breathing in a variety of ways, the diaphragm is always the most important breathing muscle. Using the diaphragm's elasticity to breathe properly is crucial in order to achieve a successful stretch as well as any other form of movement.

The depth and capacity that can be achieved through breathing efficiently is so wide that someone practising Method Putkisto should have an open mind, and explore and work often on the possibilities of the breath.

The breathing exercises of Method Putkisto – Balloon, Rising-Sun and Half-Moon – will help you to develop an awareness of your breathing muscles, which you can then harness as you wish – in performance, relaxation, well-being, and of course as a tool for your stretches.

THE DIAPHRAGM

The diaphragm is your main breathing muscle. It is an internal muscle sitting like a parachute inside your ribcage, acting as a floor for your ribcage, and a ceiling for your stomach. It is connected to the front and sides of the lower part of your ribs and to the spine in your lower back. The diaphragm is like a horizontal dividing line in your torso, between your ribcage and abdominal cavity. Its movement is partly voluntary, partly involuntary, thus it is also the dividing line between consciously and unconsciously controlled movements in your body. For instance, it is an impossibility to control the heartbeat, whereas it is possible to control the diaphragm. The diaphragm is rarely used to its full potential, which is commonly due to tight chest muscles and lack of postural support. This causes the ribcage to sink down, leading to a loss of waistline. Conversely, using the diaphragm properly forms a foundation for postural support.

When you breathe in, the diaphragm contracts, pushing down on the abdominal cavity and allowing air to move into and fill the lungs. When you breathe out, the diaphragm is relaxing, moving up towards the ribs. This recovery movement releases the air from your lungs. The sign of isolated diaphragm breathing is that no other muscles assist the breathing, as is the case when you sleep. The diaphragm is both rising and falling within the ribcage. Each rise physically lifts your ribs because the diaphragm is moving up inside the ribcage like a newly opened parachute. This action releases the air from your lungs. This is what you want to achieve.

Learning about the function of the diaphragm provides you with the means to use it more efficiently. The potential of the diaphragm is far greater than has been generally understood in physical training. Its use is crucial for efficient cardiovascular exercise or for singing, and you can learn to use it for relaxing your body during stressful situations.

Method Putkisto offers you three different techniques of breathing.

- Balloon Breathing

- Rising-Sun Breathing

- Half-Moon Breathing

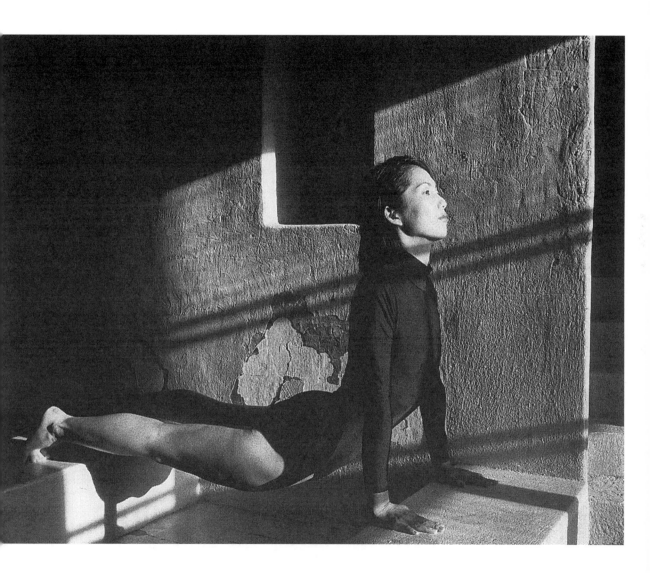

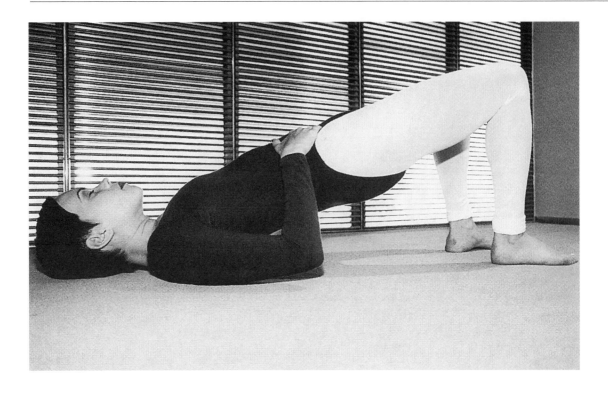

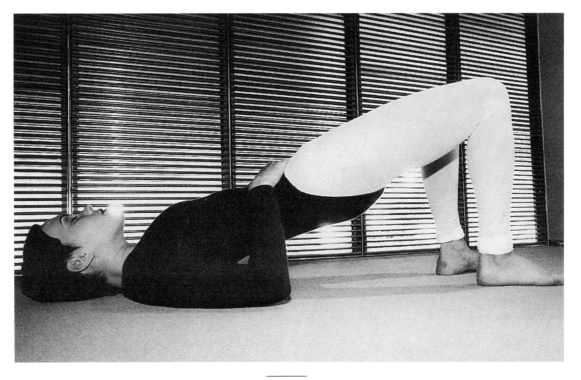

BALLOON BREATHING

Balloon breathing is a practical way of *isolating your diaphragm* and getting in touch with its action. Balloon breathing comprises the diaphragm's movement towards your pelvis during inhalation and its passive recovery rising action when air is released.

1. Lie down on your back with your knees bent. Position your feet so that your heels and knees are the same width apart as your hips, weight slightly towards the feet. Have your hands by your sides on the floor.

2. Lift your pelvis 5-13 cm (2-5 in) off the floor by tilting your tailbone towards your navel. Release your chest and solar plexus area, dropping the weight towards the base of your ribs between your shoulderblades.

Note: This position provides resistance to the contraction of the diaphragm when you breathe in. When you breathe out, the 'downhill slope' assists in the passive recovery of your diaphragm.

3. Breathe in through your nose, visualising the movement of your diaphragm down towards your pelvis, and pulling the air into your lungs. Allow the pressure of the inbreath to bring your abdomen, including your lower abdomen, out like a balloon.

Note: Be sure this occurs as a result of the diaphragm movement and not the abdominal muscles.

4. Exhale by opening your mouth and releasing the contraction of your diaphragm. This allows the air to puff out from your lungs, your stomach to fall towards the back of your ribs, and your diaphragm to recover back through your centreline.

Note: The amount of air passively released from your lungs is a measure of your diaphragm's current level of elasticity. Do not be alarmed if this action seems hard to achieve. This is a sign that you are not using your main breathing muscle effectively. As a matter of fact this is quite common, especially if there is a postural misalignment. A good deal of development is available through specific strengthening exercises as follows.

STRENGTHENING THE DIAPHRAGM

1. Repeat the balloon-breathing action, but this time press your hands in and up on to your solar plexus area underneath your breast bone. This creates an additional resistance for the diaphragm as you breathe and the pressure forces it to become stronger. Repeat the outbreath as above. DELAY after each breath in and out.

RISING-SUN BREATHING

This type of breathing is designed to get you in touch with the *upper part of your lungs.*

1. Lie on your back on the floor with a small pillow placed under your head if needed. Slightly tilt the chin down, creating a space between the top vertebrae of your spine and head, and naturally lengthening your neck.

Note: At the back of the neck feel the natural curve inward of the vertebrae, which mirrors the slightly inward curve of the lower back.

2. Place one hand on your chest, fingers up, and the other on the back of your neck, fingers reaching towards the middle of the shoulderblade area in order to focus on the upper part of your lungs. (You can remove your hands once the focus is clear.)

3. In this position breathe in through your nose, allowing your breastbone (sternum) to lift and expand as your lungs fill. DELAY. Then breathe out by allowing the ribs to soften and relax into the flow. Allow a DELAY before your next inhalation.

Note: As the lungs empty, softening of the ribs will occur naturally. You do not have to press the ribs down. Be aware of completely emptying the upper part of the lungs. You might be holding some breath in your chest. Only after fully emptying your lungs, can you fill them to a greater capacity. This will also eventually allow the area between your shoulderblades to expand as you breathe in.

If you find it difficult to inhale and exhale deeply there is too much tension in the upper back.

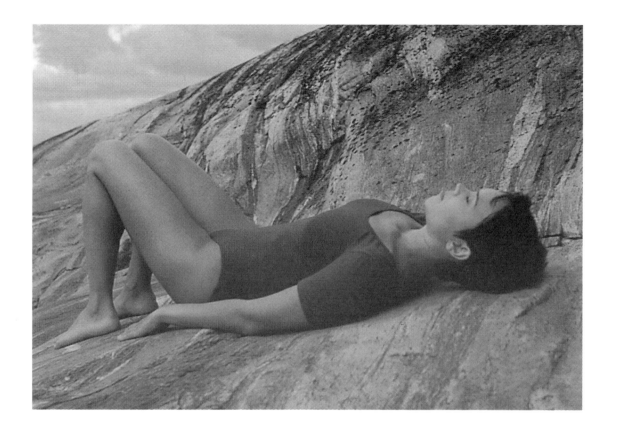

HALF-MOON BREATHING

This breathing is designed to put you in touch with the *lower parts of your lungs.* It also teaches you efficient diaphragm breathing without allowing your stomach to balloon out. Half-Moon Breathing requires engagement of your abdominal corset.

1. Choose a comfortable position, either sitting or lying down. If lying down, drop your weight toward the back of your ribs and pelvis. Place your hands on the sides and lower part of your ribcage. Keep your upper body and shoulders relaxed.

2. Breathe in. Allow your ribs to expand *sideways* against your hands, while maintaining a still centrepoint. (See Terminology, page 18.)

3. Once you have reached a deep inhalation, DELAY.

Note: After your delay you may choose to expand the pressure with a bit more inhalation.

4. Gradually breathe out through your mouth, streamlining your exhalation with the resistance of your lips.

5. As you breathe out your diaphragm will lift. Simultaneously, engage your abdominal corset to squeeze more air out of your lungs. DELAY.

Note: The lift of the diaphragm will also create a lift in your lower abdominals. Since your abdominals are your breathing muscles, they will engage if you breathe out efficiently. This requires you to maintain your centreline.

6. Repeat the breath in. This time softly engage your abdominal corset to maintain your centrepoint. Control your abdominal corset throughout the breathing as you continue, placing an emphasis on the contraction of the corset with each outbreath.

USING BREATHING IN DEEP STRETCHING

Maximise your stretch by timing your inbreath and outbreath: the momentum of your diaphragm. Between each change in its direction there is a fraction of a DELAY. Controlling your diaphragm at these moments and delaying the next inhalation allows you to move deeper into your stretch.

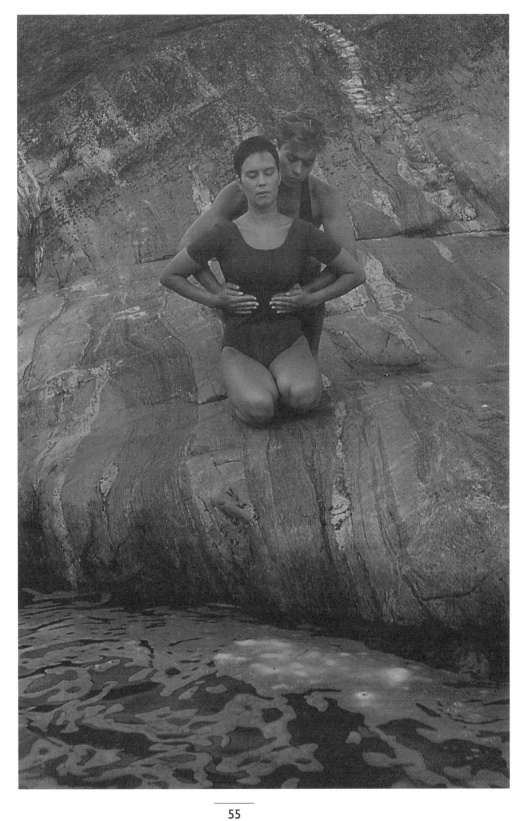

2

WARMING UP

The following warm-up is a good way to prepare you for stretching as well as centring you before going through the exercises. This will help you to be more aware of your centre as you work. If you would like to warm your muscles further before stretching, try some bicycling or gentle aerobic exercises.

1. Lie down on your back, with legs bent and feet flat on the floor. Drop your weight on to the back of your pelvis and back of your ribs. Tilt your pelvis ten times, initiating the movement from your tailbone up (towards your navel) and down (away from your navel). Relax your weight on it. Establish your centreline.

Note: Engage your 'pelvic floor' muscles (see Terminology, page 17).

2. Return to your starting position. Bring your knees up to your chest. Place your hands on your knees and lift your elbows to the sides, away from your body. Moving your legs with your hands, hug them close enough into your chest to create a gentle stretch in your lower back. Move slowly enough to give yourself time to feel the weight on the lower back. Return to the starting position.

3. Go through each of the three breathing techniques. Begin with Balloon Breathing, move to Rising-Sun and then focus on Half-Moon Breathing.

Note: Once you feel you have been able to find a nice flow for your breathing, stay with Half-Moon Breathing as you work through your warm-up.

4. Clasp your hands behind your head. Use your abdominals and Half-Moon Breathing to do small sit-ups. Lift your shoulders off the floor by engaging your *abdominal corset*. Breathe out as you lift. Holding the lift in your shoulders, continue breathing out. Allow your centrepoint to sink down toward the back of your ribs. Due to the

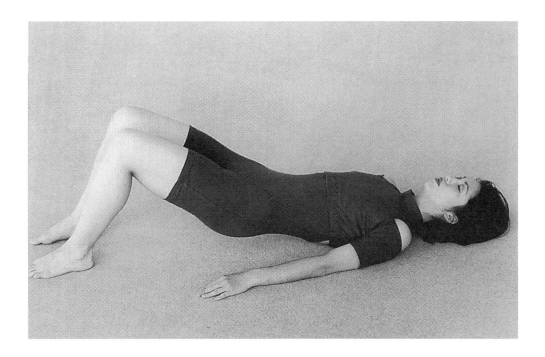

breathing, feel the lift also in your lower abdominals.

Breathe in as you lower, maintaining your centreline. Repeat five to ten times.

Note: Create opposition for your sit-up by keeping enough weight on your tailbone. (See Terminology, Hip Flexor and Abdominal Corset.)

Note: To help you get the correct starting position without engaging your neck, you can use a firm pillow under your upper back.

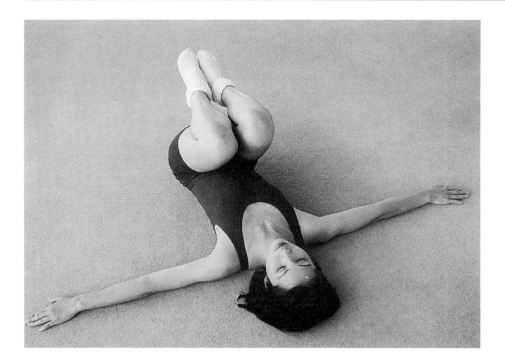

5. Return to your starting position. Extend your arms straight out from your sides, on the floor, palms down.

* Breathe in using Half-Moon Breathing, and roll your bent knees over to your right and look to the left (opposition of movement).

* Breathe out, emphasising the contraction of your abdominal corset as you return your knees to their centre position.

* Repeat to the left side, breathing in and looking to the right. Breathe out as you return to your centre. Repeat the exercise three times on each side.

Note: Take notice of the diagonal use of your abdominal corset.

Note: If you find you are arching your back, make the movements smaller.

6. Roll over on to your stomach. Bend your arms and place your hands on the floor in line with your shoulders. Align your head with your spine. Curve your chest off the floor by extending your arms, and lift your chin slightly up. Breathe in using either Rising-Sun or Balloon Breathing. During the outbreath feel a slight stretch in your abdominal area. Keep your lower back and buttocks relaxed. Lower your chest to the floor by bending your arms.

7. Use your hands to push yourself back on to your knees and then on to your heels. Curl your toes under for a stretch. Now use your hands once again to push back on to your feet.

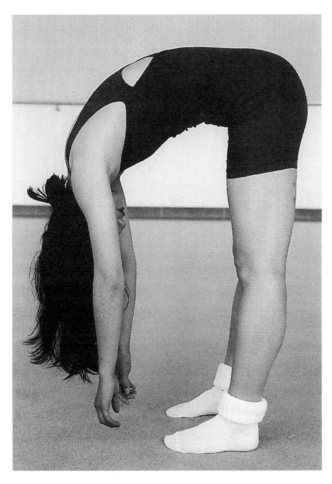

8. Keep your head down. Begin to straighten your legs, but if needed keep the knees slightly bent and breathe in. During the outbreath, roll up through your spine while engaging your abdominal corset, initiating the movement from your tailbone by tilting it towards your navel. Keep your buttocks relaxed.

9. Link your hands behind your back. Press your shoulderblades together. Extend your arms down towards the floor and lift your chest. Release your arms.

10. Extend your arms above your head and clasp your hands together. Look upwards, allowing your chest to lift. Breathe in using Rising-Sun. Breathe out. Once you have emptied your lungs, lower your arms, find your centreline and begin your stretching session.

3

WAISTLINE AND ABDOMINALS

1. Bow Stretch

2. Floor Arch

3. Triangle Stretch

MAIN EFFECTS

Increases length of waist, shapes waist, pulls the stomach in, increases the use of the diaphragm, relieves tension in lower back, and reduces cellulite.

MUSCLE TARGETS

Quadratus Lumborum, Iliopsoas, Transversus and Rectus Abdominis, Internal and External Obliques.

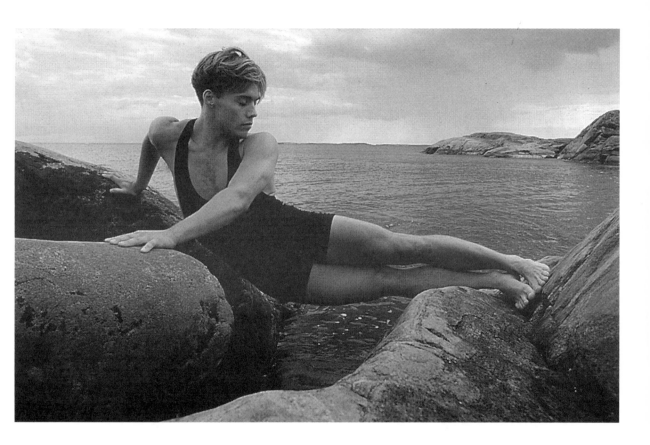

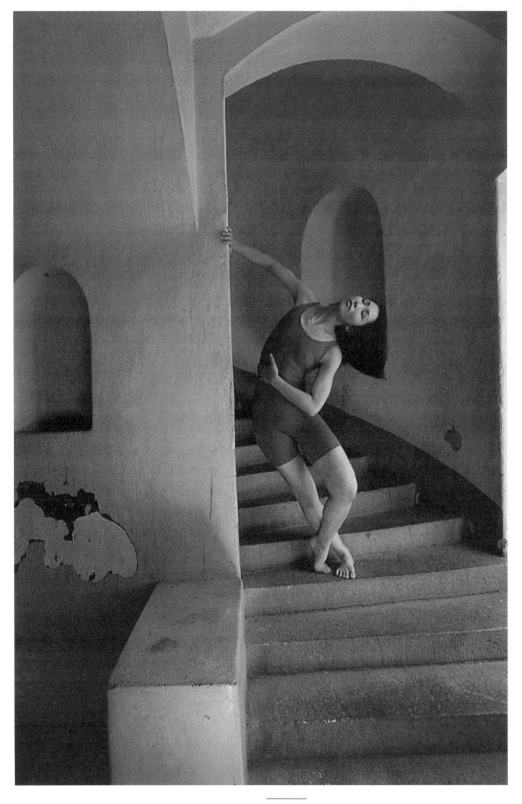

BOW STRETCH

POSITION

Stand right side to a wall. Place the heel of your left foot over or on top of your right foot. Lift the right elbow upwards rotating it from the shoulder. Place the palm of your hand against the wall at a height which feels comfortable. Drop your head towards your left shoulder. Place your left hand on the right side of your lower ribcage.

NOTE

The rotation of the elbow opens the space between your ribcage and pelvis. The placement of your left hand will clarify the focus for your breathing as well as the stretch. (You can move it elsewhere while you stretch, if needed.)

STEPS

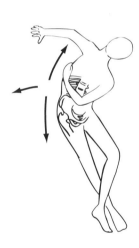

* Focus on your waistline and on increasing the space between your pelvis and ribcage.

* Create a 'bow' shape by bending your supporting leg and arm.

* Breathe in to expand the side you are stretching.

* Create the stretch as you breathe out and the rise of the diaphragm lifts your ribs away from your pelvis.

* DELAY, and then further separate your ribs from your pelvis by dropping your weight towards your waistline. Be careful not to lean on your hand.

* Continue the stretch with the flow of your breathing. Slowly extend your right leg, working against your groundpoint. Keep your tailbone towards your navel.

NOTE

Since this is a strong stretch to begin with, try to find an easier way for yourself – the target is to lift the lowest rib (and thus the ribcage) away from your pelvis. Look at the Standing Lunge on page 75.

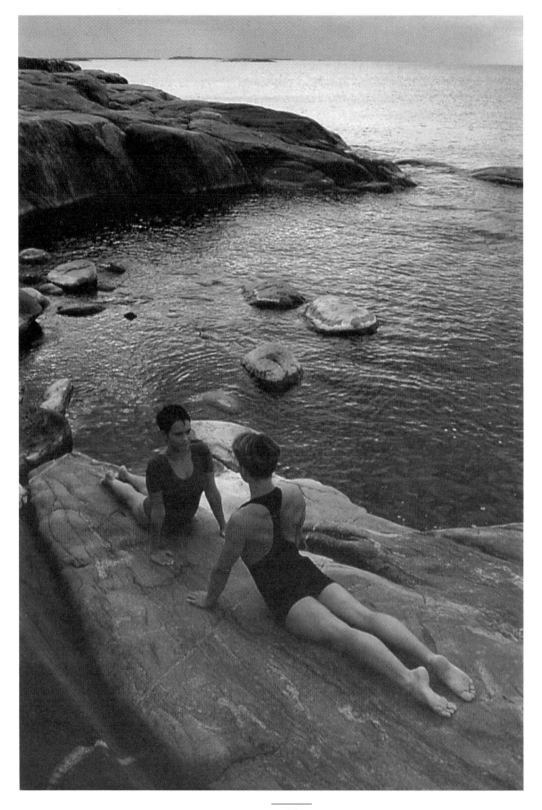

FLOOR ARCH

POSITION

Lie face down on the floor and extend your legs fully. Bend your arms and place your hands on the floor in line with your shoulders. Lift your abdominals towards your spine. Relax your lower back. Tilt the pelvis by turning your tailbone towards your navel. Keep your buttocks relaxed. Lift your chest by extending your arms. Rotate your shoulders back.

STEPS

* Focus on the abdominal muscles.

* Breathe in, using Balloon Breathing.

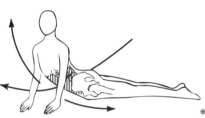

* Create the stretch with your breath as you breathe out. Allowing your weight to drop to the top of your thighs acts as your ground point. Feel the stretch increasing in your lower abdominal muscles during the DELAY of your breathing.

* Continue the stretch, moving into Rising-Sun Breathing. Engage your abdominal corset and lift your chest and chin. Keep the head upright, maintaining the length in the back of your neck. Keep the shoulderblades down.

NOTE

You may modify this stretch by lifting your chest with your hands holding on to a staircase or a barre. By flexing your toes, rather than extending them, you can create an even deeper stretch.

TRIANGLE STRETCH

You may have to begin this stretch by working on lengthening both your front thighs as well as your hip flexors until they are long enough for you to be able to reach the position described below. (See Basic Lunge, page 71, and Lightening Stretch, Angle 1, page 85.)

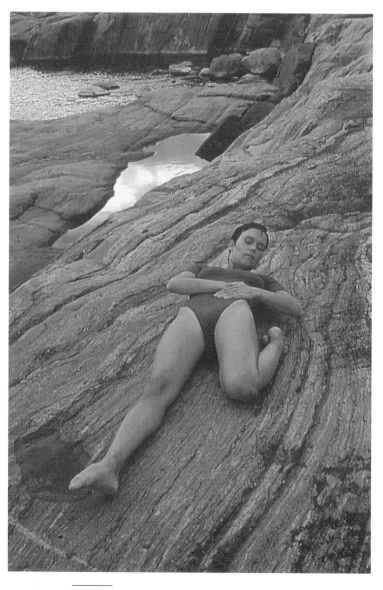

POSITION   Sit on the floor with your left leg bent at the knee, tucked to the side and parallel to the right leg. Rotate it inward from the hip joint. The right leg is extended and relaxed. Lean back by supporting your body weight on your hands, fingers pointing forward, or bend the elbows and support your weight on your elbows.

STEPS   * Focus on the muscles in the front of the thigh of your bent leg, aiming to stretch your lower abdominal muscles.

            * Breathe in using Balloon Breathing. During the outbreath, start to lower yourself down on to your elbows and then on to your back.

            * Create the stretch by moving to the Diaphragm-Strengthening Breath (see page 51). Place your hands on your abdomen. As you breathe in, resist the pressure of the breathing with your hands.

            * As you breathe out, pull the abdominals gently down and then upwards towards your ribs. Tilt your tailbone up towards your navel, keep your buttocks relaxed. Feel the stretch in the very lower part of your abdominals.

            * DELAY. Take your time before the next inbreath.

NOTE   To ease the stretch a little, you may have to use a pillow under your lower back.

VARIATION   The position of this stretch may be modified by taking the same position but with both legs bent under, or with the foot of the extended leg on top of the knee of the bent leg.

4

PELVIS AND BUTTOCKS

1. Basic Lunge

2. Sitting Lunge

3. Standing Lunge

4. Rotation

MAIN EFFECTS

Changes the tilt of the pelvis, opens the lower back and lifts the buttock line, increases circulation, and reduces cellulite.

MUSCLE TARGETS

Gluteus Maximus, Gluteus Medius, Hip flexors, Upper Rectus Femoris.

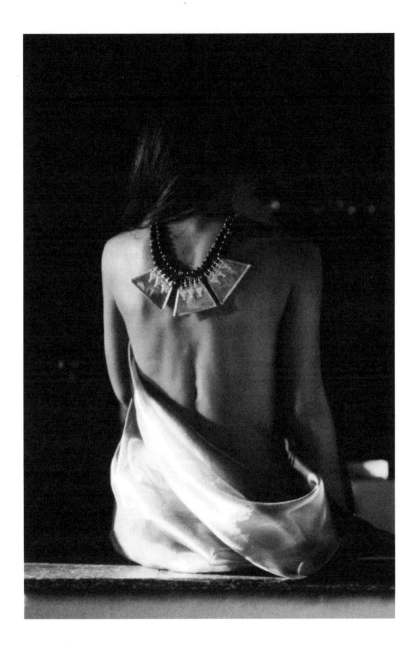

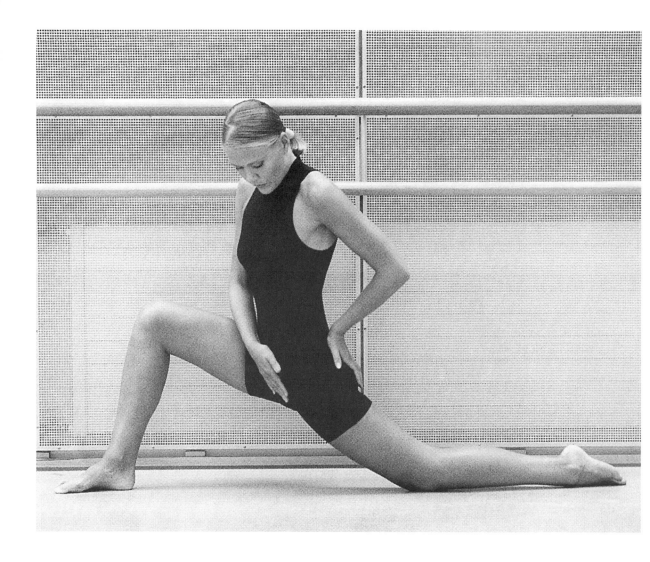

BASIC LUNGE

POSITION
Kneel on the floor. Bend the right leg creating a 90-degree angle in front of your body. Stabilise the foot flat on the floor. Find your centreline. Extend your back leg fully. Stay upright with your chest lifted. Tilt your tailbone towards your navel. Rotate your back leg from your hip joint slightly inwards.

NOTE
You can have supports on either side if you like. These you can use to ease up the pressure on the pelvic area, by transferring some of your weight to your arm or arms.

STEPS

* Focus on the deep muscles of the hip area (see Hip Flexor, page 17). To clarify this focus, place your left hand on the front of the hip of the extended leg, and the other on your right buttock (slightly above your tailbone).

* Breathe in using Balloon Breathing.

* Move your front hand on to the support. Create the stretch at the end of the outbreath (DELAY). Apply more body weight gradually through your pelvis to increase the stretch.You can press with the hand on your buttocks to help the forward movement of the tailbone towards your navel.

* Continue the stretch with the flow of your breathing.

NOTE
Due to the depth of the muscles, it is important during the outbreath to feel the lift in the lower abdominal area as the diaphragm is moving up towards the ribcage.

NOTE
Using Half-Moon Breathing will access a different way of experiencing the stretch.

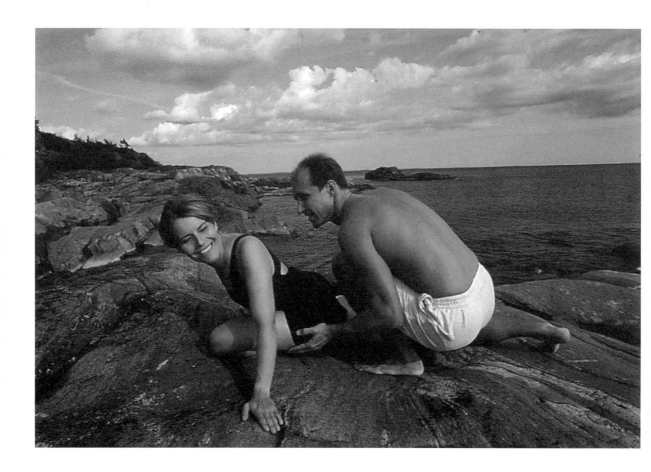

SITTING LUNGE

POSITION

Get into the basic lunge position, with the left leg bent in front, the other extended behind. Place your hands to the sides for support. Turn the knee of your front leg to the left on the floor. Move your foot to the right towards your centre line, and sit on your left buttock. Keep the back leg extended behind you, and turn it slightly in from the top of the leg. Move your pelvis into an upright position. Lean slightly forward, bending your arms.

STEPS

* Focus on the deeper muscles of the buttock, the sitting bone area, on the left side.

* Use Half-Moon Breathing to open the lower back.

* Create the stretch while breathing out. Bend your arms to apply additional weight through the part of the buttock you are working on.

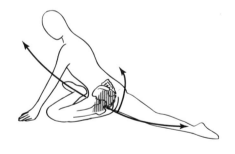

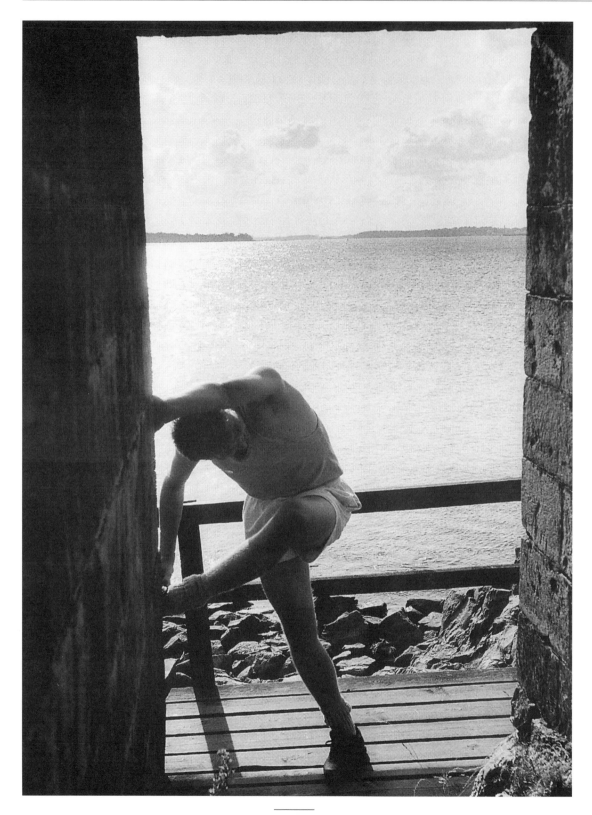

STANDING LUNGE

POSITION

Standing beside a wall or supporting surface, lift and bend your left leg up in front of you at waist height. Rest your foot and bent leg on the wall or surface and drop the knee to the left. Turn the standing leg in at the hip and keep your pelvis facing forward. Place your hands on the support, and curve the upper body over your leg. Control your weight with your hands.

STEPS

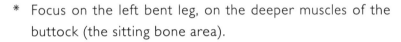
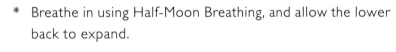
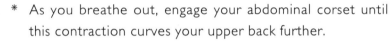

* Focus on the left bent leg, on the deeper muscles of the buttock (the sitting bone area).

* Breathe in using Half-Moon Breathing, and allow the lower back to expand.

* As you breathe out, engage your abdominal corset until this contraction curves your upper back further.

* Create the stretch with the opposition of movement. Bend your right, standing leg and turn your left knee further towards the floor. You will feel the stretch in your buttocks. Keep your sitting bones at the original height.

* Deepen the stretch by rotating your torso towards your left, bent leg, and repeat the bend of your right leg. Transfer more of your body weight on to the right, standing leg.

NOTE

Take your time with this stretch. Since the muscles are deep and strong, it may take 10-20 seconds before you can even *feel* them.

NOTE

You can also use this stretch to mobilise your waistline and open up your lower back instead of the Bow Stretch (see page 63). Lift your lowest rib away from the hip, and tilt your ribcage further away from the bent leg instead of the buttocks. Focus on the space between your lowest rib and hip – on the lower back.

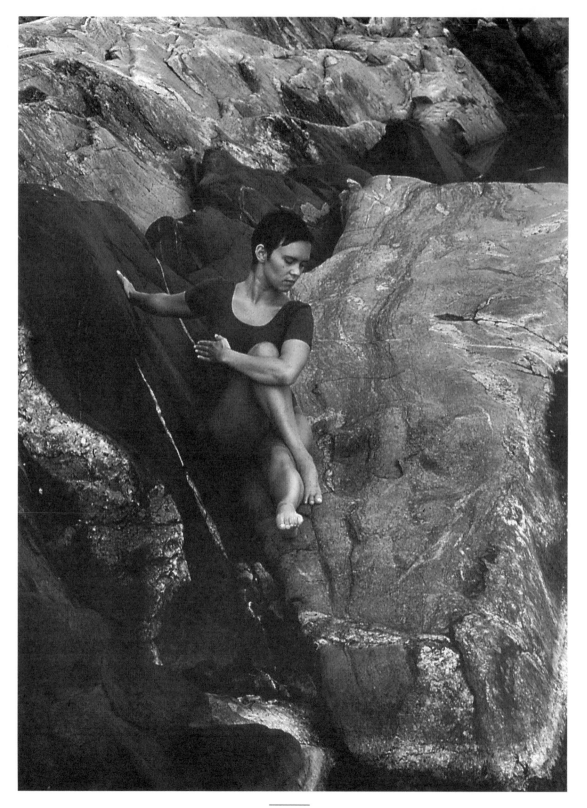

ROTATION

POSITION

Sit with your back half an arm's length from a wall, your legs out in front of you. Bend your right leg and cross it over your left. Clasp your right knee with your left arm, and press it against your centrepoint. Place your right hand at shoulder level on to the wall behind you. Keeping your back upright, turn your torso towards the right. Use the support of the right hand on the wall to further lift the torso up and around its centre. Turn your focus to the right and lock your abdominal corset.

NOTE

Keep both your sitting bones on the floor.

STEPS

* Focus on the lower back area and deeper buttock muscles.

* Breathe in using Half-Moon Breathing.

* As you breathe out, rotate your torso towards the right. Create the opposition of movement with your right hand on the wall to further lift the torso up and around your centrepoint.

NOTE

As this is a relatively contained position, take the opportunity to feel the opening of the lower back area created by the breathing. Depending on your flexibility, however, this stretch may travel further up and around the back.

NOTE

If the position of this stretch is uncomfortable, do not cross the one leg over the other. The extended leg can also be slightly bent.

LEGS

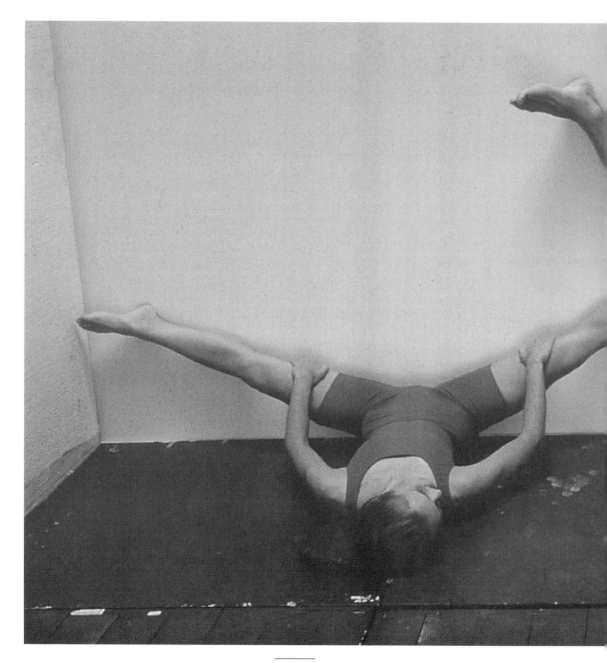

Begin with the Basic Lunge (see page 71). Focus your stretch on the upper part of your thigh until the muscle length allows you to tilt your pelvis correctly for all the following Lunges. Progress to the Lightening Stretch, Angle 1 or the Rotation Lunge, Angle 1. Angles 2-3 are for more defined work towards shaping your thighs (see also Triangle Stretch, page 66).

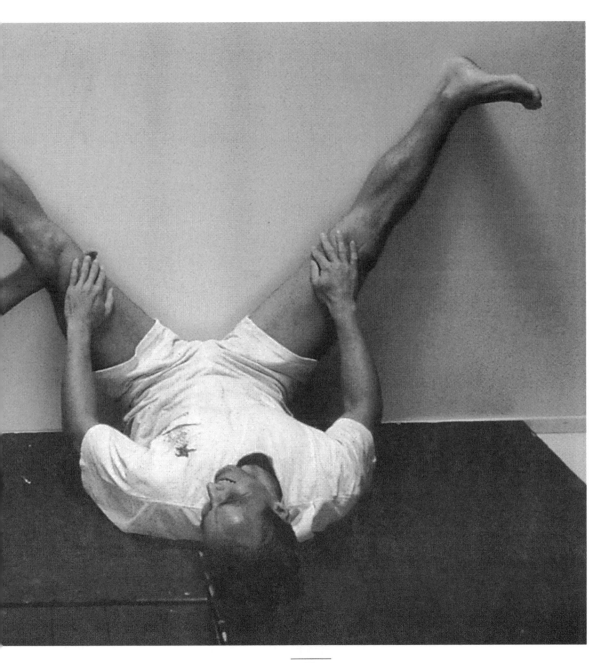

5

FRONT OF THIGHS

1. Rotation Lunge, Angles 1-3
2. Lightening Stretch, Angles 1-3

MAIN EFFECTS

Changes the shape of the front of your legs, adjusts the tilt of the pelvis.

MUSCLE TARGETS

Rectus Femoris, Vastus Lateralis, Vastus Intermedius, Vastus Medialis, Sartorius, Quadriceps Femoris.

ROTATION LUNGE
Angle I

POSITION

Assume the Basic Lunge. Use an appropriate support at chest height, and something soft under your knee. Bring your right foot closer to your pelvis. Bend the knee of your left extended leg, and use the left arm to slowly pull the heel toward your buttock. Transfer your weight forward, away from your knee. Keep the left elbow up and fingers pointing down, grasping the toes.

STEPS

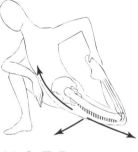

* Focus on the middle of your front thigh.

* Use Balloon Breathing.

* Once you feel the muscle, lean further forward over your supporting foot. Create a deeper stretch by slowly bringing the foot of the left leg even closer to your buttocks. Keep tilting your tailbone towards your navel.

NOTE

Be sure that you do not contract the hip flexor at the same time. The front thigh muscles have a strong biting point.

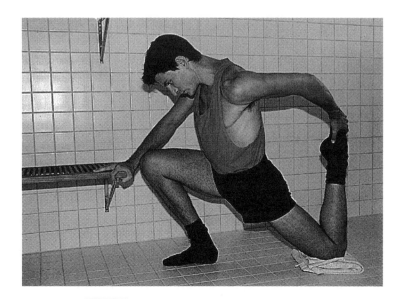

ROTATION LUNGE
Angle 2

POSITION

Assume the basic lunge position. Repeat as above in Angle 1, but keep the left elbow up and press the palm of the hand against the *inside* of the left foot.

STEPS

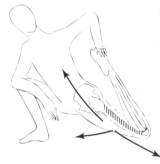

* Focus on the *outside* of the front of your thigh.

* Use Balloon Breathing.

* Once you feel the muscle responding, lean further forward over your supporting foot. Create a deeper stretch by slowly pushing the foot of the left leg away to the side and then bring it slowly towards your buttocks. Keep tilting your tailbone towards your navel.

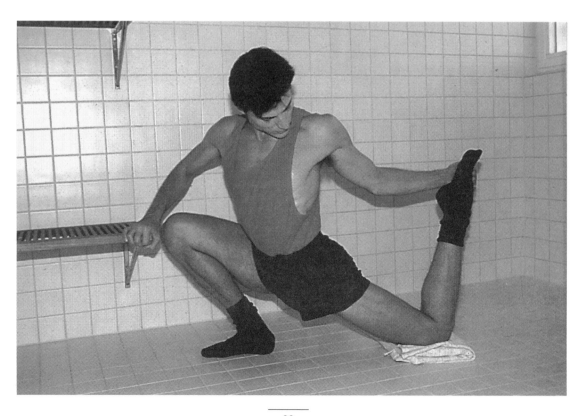

ROTATION LUNGE
Angle 3

POSITION

Assume the Basic Lunge. Repeat as above in Angle 1. This time press with your *right hand* towards the *outside of your left foot*. Bring your foot with your right hand towards the *inside of your buttocks*. At the same time turn your torso towards your right foot.

STEPS

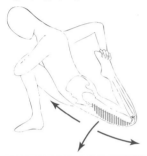

* Focus on the *inside* of the front of your thigh.

* Use Balloon Breathing.

* Once you feel the muscle responding, create a deeper stretch by slowly pulling the heel of your right leg closer towards your buttocks, feeling the stretch inside the front thigh.

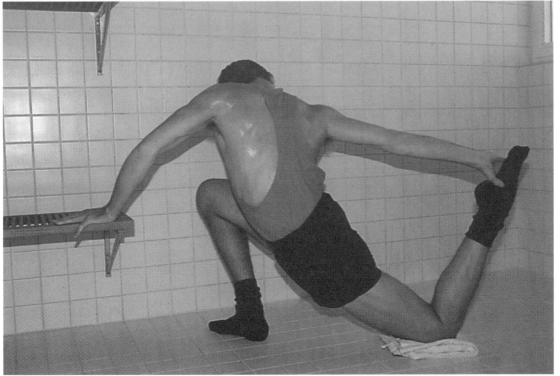

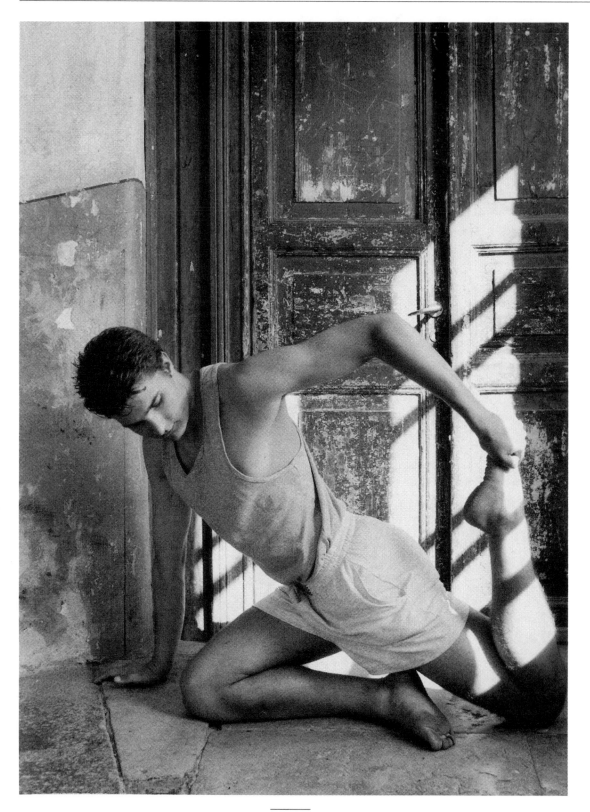

LIGHTENING STRETCH
Angles 1-3

NOTE

These stretches are variations on Rotation Lunges, Angles 1-3, for those who may have tight hip flexors and therefore find it difficult to maintain a Basic Lunge.

POSITION

Kneel, and extend the left leg back. Use your arms for support. Rest on the front thigh and bend the left leg above the knee. Use your left arm for Angle 1 and Angle 2. Use your opposite arm for Angle 3.

STEPS

* These are the same as the corresponding Rotation Lunges, Angles 1-3.

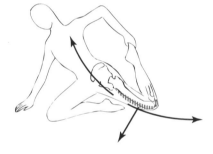

6

INNER THIGHS

1. Standing V

2. Sitting V

3. Lying V

MAIN EFFECTS

The positioning of your pelvis and shape of the buttocks.

MUSCLE TARGETS

Adductor Brevis, Adductor Longus, Adductor Magnus, Gracilis.

STANDING V

POSITION   Stand next to a hip-high surface or beside a wall. Extend your right leg out to the side and lift it on to a suitable level of the surface. Maintain your weight on your left, supporting leg. Place your left hand on the top of your left knee and extend the right arm along the right leg. Bend the left leg and rotate the right leg outwards. Assume the Flat-Back Pelvic Tilt (see page 42).

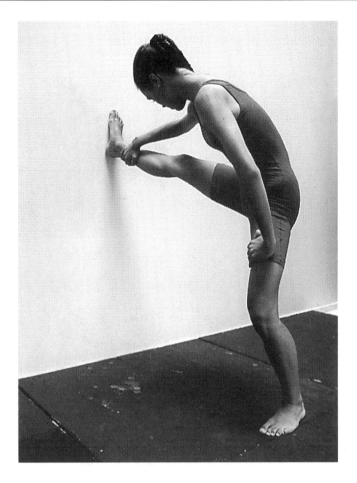

STEPS

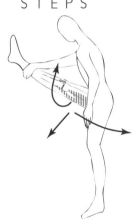

* Focus on the inner thigh muscles. Separate the top of your right leg from the pubic and sitting bones. Find your centreline.

* Breathe in using Half-Moon Breathing, and bend your supporting leg.

* Create the stretch as you breathe out, slowly straightening your left, supporting leg, working towards the ground point.

* Once you clearly feel the muscles of the inner thigh, apply body weight on them for a deeper stretch.

NOTE

Try turning out the right leg at the hip by using the deeper buttock muscles. This action will further separate the top of your leg from your pelvis.

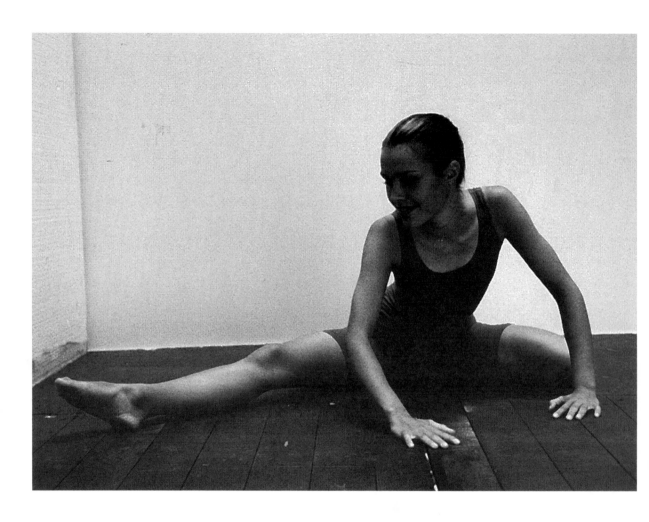

SITTING V

POSITION

Sit on the floor. Tuck your left leg underneath your pelvis, extending the right leg out to the side. Place your hands in front of you and lift your weight off the floor. Tilt your tailbone away from your navel, following with your torso. Lean forward. If needed, place a small pillow underneath your right knee to lift it.

NOTE

Do not move the weight too far away from your ground point.

STEPS

* Focus on the inner thigh muscles.

* Breathe in using Balloon Breathing.

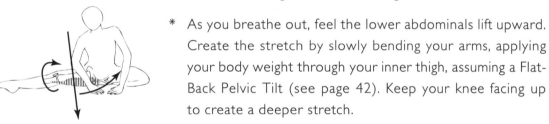

* As you breathe out, feel the lower abdominals lift upward. Create the stretch by slowly bending your arms, applying your body weight through your inner thigh, assuming a Flat-Back Pelvic Tilt (see page 42). Keep your knee facing up to create a deeper stretch.

NOTE

You can also place the right foot towards the wall, toes facing up.

LYING V

POSITION

Lie flat on your back with your pelvis and legs, feet up, against a wall. Open your legs to a V position and rotate the legs outward from the hip joint. Keep the sitting bones at a 90-degree angle with the wall. Relax your weight on to the back of your pelvis.

STEPS

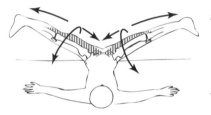

* Focus on the inner thigh muscles.

* Breathe in using Half-Moon Breathing.

* As you breathe out, lift your lower abdominal muscles but anchor your tailbone to the floor. Rotate the legs slightly further outward.

* Take a substantial amount of time with this stretch (5-8 minutes), and remember to relax.

NOTE

As your stretch continues, you may apply additional weight by placing your hands on the inner thighs and gently pressing downwards, according to what your range of rotation will allow.

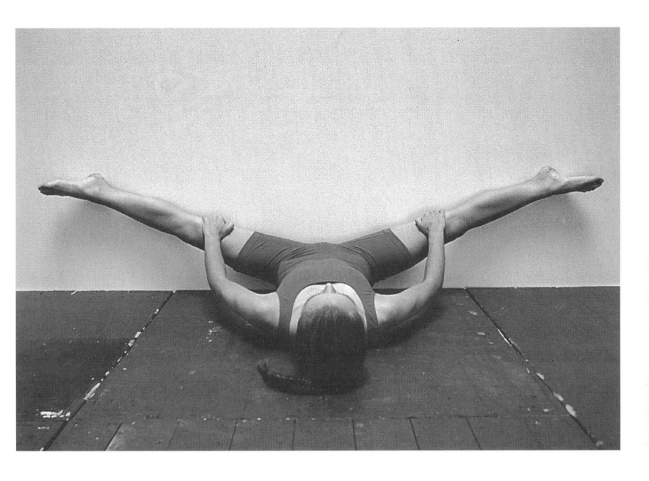

7

BACK OF THIGHS

1. L-Pull

2. V-Tilt

MAIN EFFECTS

Lifts buttocks, changes the tilt of your pelvis and your back. Releases lower back tension, and connects leg muscles.

MUSCLE TARGETS

Hamstrings (Semimembranosus, Semitendinosus, Biceps Femoris).

L-PULL

POSITION   Stand beside a waist-high surface. Extend your left leg and lift your heel on to the surface. Soften the knee. Bend it enough to enable you to assume the Flat-Back Pelvic Tilt (see page 42).

NOTE   The tilt of the tailbone will separate the top of the leg from the sitting bone.

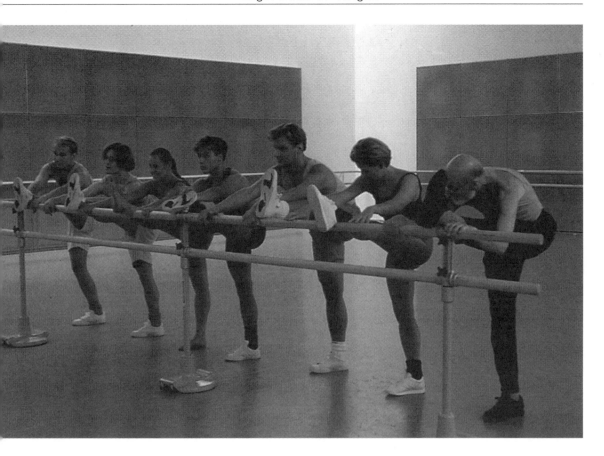

STEPS

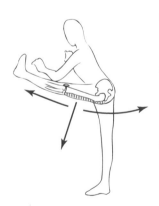

* Focus on your hamstrings.

* Breathe in using Half-Moon Breathing. Bend the right supporting leg.

* As you breathe out, create the stretch by slowly straightening the right leg and, working towards the ground point, transferring the weight of your torso forward.

* Once you are able to feel the stretch, deepen it by repeating the above, and gradually applying more body weight through the back of your thigh muscles.

NOTE

Push your heel into the floor for a controlled straightening of the leg. Continue to tilt your tailbone away from your navel. As the hamstring lengthens you may gradually decrease the bend in your left knee.

V-TILT

(See also V-Tilt in Calves and Feet.)

POSITION
Stand facing the wall. Place the toes of your left foot against the wall with your heel on the floor. Place the right leg one stride behind the left. Lean your body forward to support your body weight with your hands on the floor. Soften the left knee by bending it slightly, enough to ensure the Flat-Back Pelvic Tilt (see page 42). This will separate the leg from the sitting bone. Relax your neck and drop your head sideways and down, avoiding the wall.

STEPS

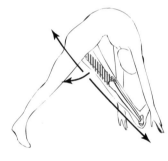

* Focus on the muscles of the back of your leg and back of your knee.

* Breathe in using Half-Moon Breathing, and bend your right supporting leg, lifting the heel up.

* As you breathe out, create the stretch by straightening the right leg, applying more body weight to the muscles of the back of your thigh.

* Deepen the stretch, bending or straightening the leg behind you. As you begin to straighten it, push the heel into the floor and continue tilting your tailbone away from your navel and further lengthening the hamstring.

* Continue moving your right leg further back, and repeat the above.

NOTE   In this position you will feel a strong sensation of the nerves (see Nerve Stretch, page 41).

NOTE   The V-Tilt stretch may be preferred to the L-Pull by those who control their body weight better with their arms or find the hamstrings in the the L-Pull difficult to work on. Ease the V-Tilt by kneeling on the leg behind you.Use something soft under your knee. Keep your weight on your arms. By bending and extending your arms, you can gradually create a deep stretch.

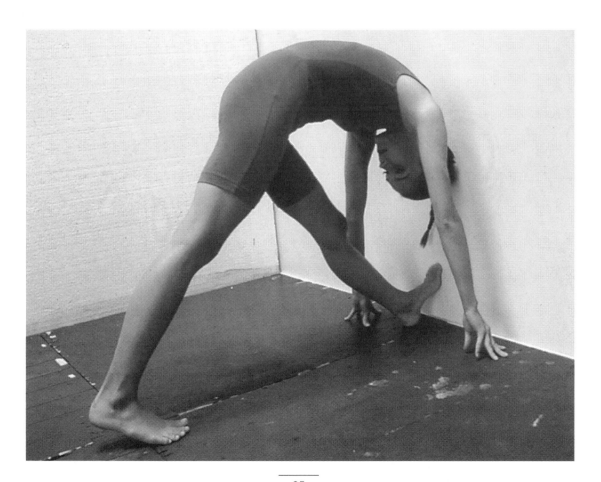

8

OUTER THIGHS

I. Outside Leg Spiral

MAIN EFFECTS:

Alters the shape of the legs, particularly their straightness.

Note: Tightness can be the result of a weakness and shortness in the deeper buttock muscles, and can cause inwardly curved legs.

MUSCLE TARGETS

Tensor Fasciae Latae.

OUTSIDE LEG SPIRAL

POSITION   Stand next to a wall or support. Extend the right leg diagonally in front of you against the wall or support. Rotate it outwards. Rotate your left supporting leg in. Lean your torso and left arm forward diagonally towards your right leg. Keep on tilting your tailbone away from your navel.

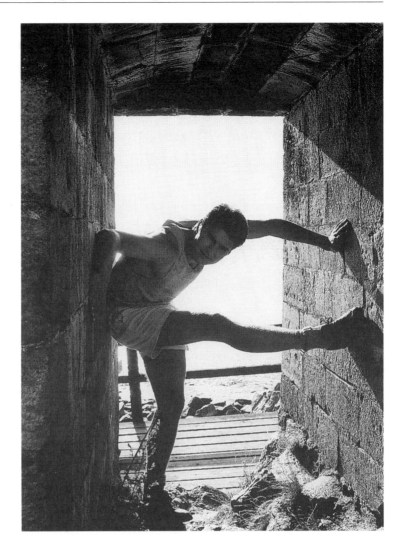

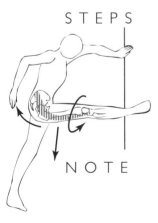

S T E P S

* Focus on the outside of your thigh.

* Breathe in, using Half-Moon Breathing.

* With your outbreath create the stretch. Slowly turn your torso to the right, leaning slightly forward. Create the stretch by giving yourself enough time to feel the stretch.

N O T E

Be careful when applying body weight. For most people this outside leg muscle is a blind spot. Using visualisation is important to connect with this muscle. Be prepared to spend at least 5 minutes stretching.

VARIATION You can do the Outside Leg Spiral stretch while kneeling. Use your arms on the floor to support the stretch. If you cannot connect to this stretch, first focus on lengthening your hamstrings and tight front muscles.

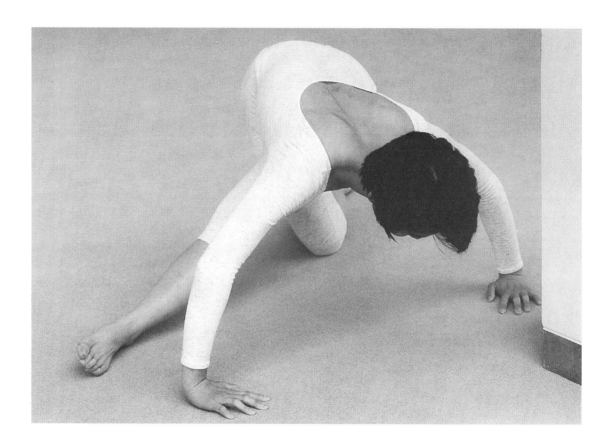

9

CALVES AND FEET

1. Full-Body Tilt

2. V-Tilt

3. Tibialis Stretch

4. Big Toe Stretch (Flexor)

5. Back of Toe Stretch (Extensor)

MAIN EFFECTS

Improves circulation of the legs, shapes the lower part the legs and knees, and slims the ankles.

MUSCLE TARGETS

Tibialis Anterior, Soleus, Gastrocnemius, Flexors, Extensors.

FULL-BODY TILT

P O S I T I O N   Stand sideways in a door frame. Flex your left foot upwards and place your toes against the frame, weight on your heel. Keep the line of your leg straight from your heel to your tailbone. Place the right foot half a stride behind the left. Relax your toes. Place your hands on the side of the door frame. Keep your torso upright and forward.

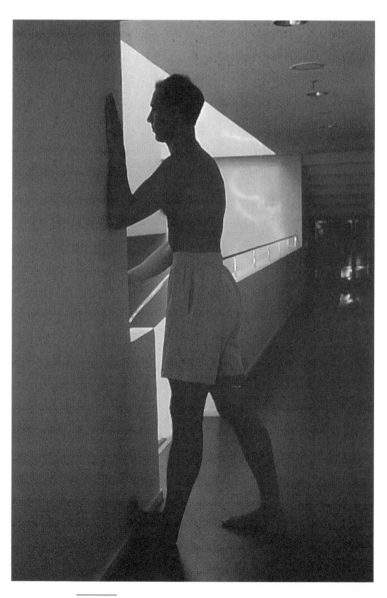

STEPS

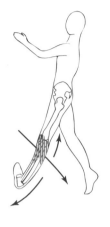

* Focus on your left calf muscles and Achilles tendon.

* Breathe in using Half-Moon Breathing.

* Breathe out and begin to lift the heel of your right foot off the floor.

* While maintaining your upright position, create the stretch by shifting your body as a whole unit towards the wall and transferring your body weight into the left calf. Use both the right leg and your arms while you pull your body forward. Keep the left leg passive.

* Try to move the toes of your left foot to help you feel the muscle connections from your toes to your calves.

VARIATION

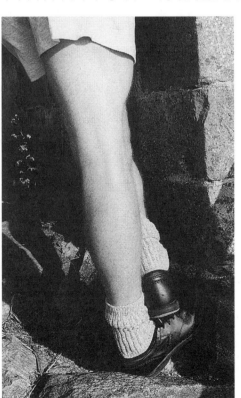

To stretch a deeper layer of the calf muscles or the Achilles tendon, begin with both knees bent. Create the stretch by first extending the left knee, working against the ground point. Once the stretch has increased you may lift the right leg off the floor and place it across the top of the left foot.

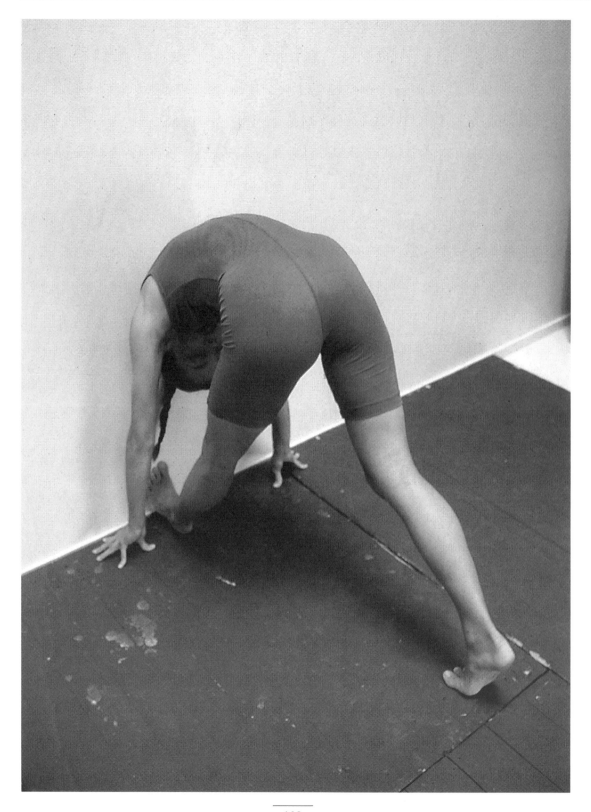

V-TILT

(See also V-Tilt in Back of Thighs.)

POSITION — Place the toes of your left foot against a wall with your heel on the floor. Place the right leg one stride behind the left. Lean your body forward and assume the Flat-Back Pelvic Tilt (see page 42). Place your hands on the floor to support your body weight. Bend the right leg and soften the left knee by bending it slightly (never lock it). Drop your head down.

NOTE — Bend the right leg enough to assume the Flat-Back Pelvic Tilt. This movement will separate the top of the leg from the sitting bone.

STEPS —

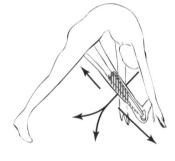

* Focus on your left calf muscles or the back of your left knee.

* Breathe in using Half-Moon Breathing. Bend the right supporting leg.

* As you breathe out, begin to straighten the right leg. Push the heel into the floor for a controlled stretch.

* As the calf begins to lengthen, you may gradually decrease the bend in your left knee and send more body weight forward.

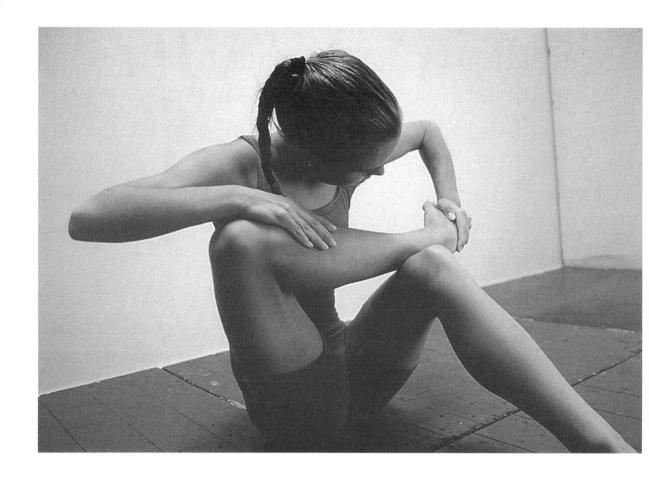

TIBIALIS STRETCH

POSITION — Sit on the floor and bend your knees. Keep your left foot flat on the floor in front of you. Pick up your right leg with your left hand and bend it over your left leg. Rest your right ankle on top of your left thigh. Grasp the bottom three toes in your left palm. Lift your left elbow 45 degrees out to the side. Keep elbow in place, back straight.

NOTE — Use a chair to sit on if it feels more comfortable for your back.

STEPS —

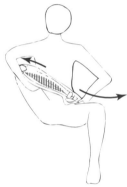

* Focus on the tibialis anterior which runs along the front of your lower leg.

* Breathe normally.

* Lean forward and down towards your body to create the stretch, at the same time pressing your toes down.

* Increase the stretch by pressing your toes down towards your body. Keep your elbow up.

BIG TOE STRETCH
(Flexor)

POSITION

Assume the Tibialis Stretch position as overleaf, except grab the big toe.

Focus on the front of your foot. Create the stretch by pressing your big toe towards your body and slightly down.

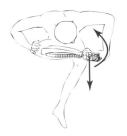

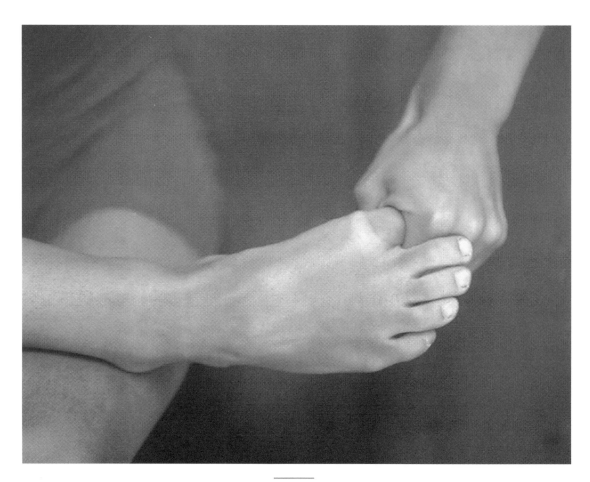

BACK OF TOE STRETCH
(Extensor)

POSITION   Kneel. Place your hands on the floor for support, fingers forwards or backwards. Tuck your toes underneath you.

STEPS

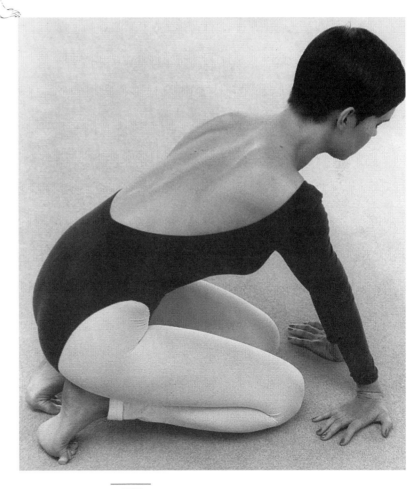

* Focus on the underneath of your toes.

* Breathe normally.

* Create the stretch by pushing the floor away with your hands, and thus applying body weight into the back of your toes.

10

BACK

1. Doorpost Stretch

2. Upside-Down Stretch

3. Staircase Stretch

4. Leg-over-Head Stretch

MAIN EFFECTS

Lifts your back, shapes your waistline, pulls your stomach in, lifts your chest, reduces tension in the back, alleviates tiredness and stabilises your arms.

MUSCLE TARGETS

Trapezius, Pectoralis Minor, Rhomboids Major and Minor, Serratus Anterior.

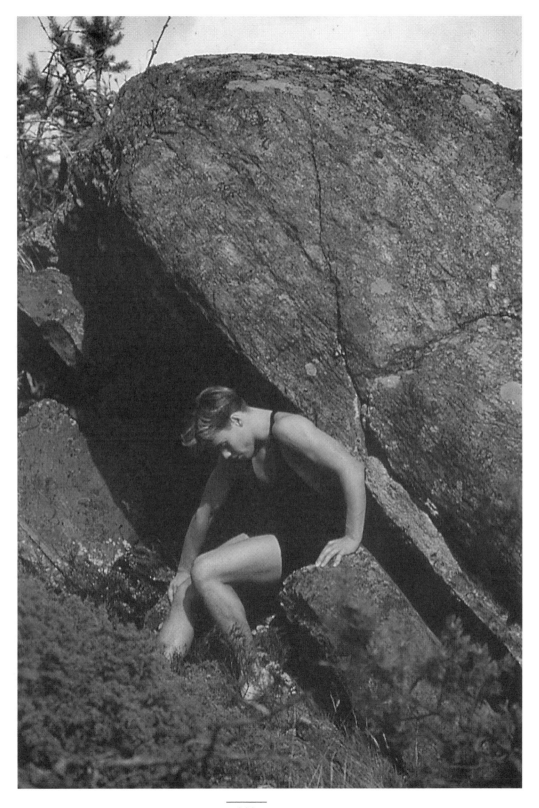

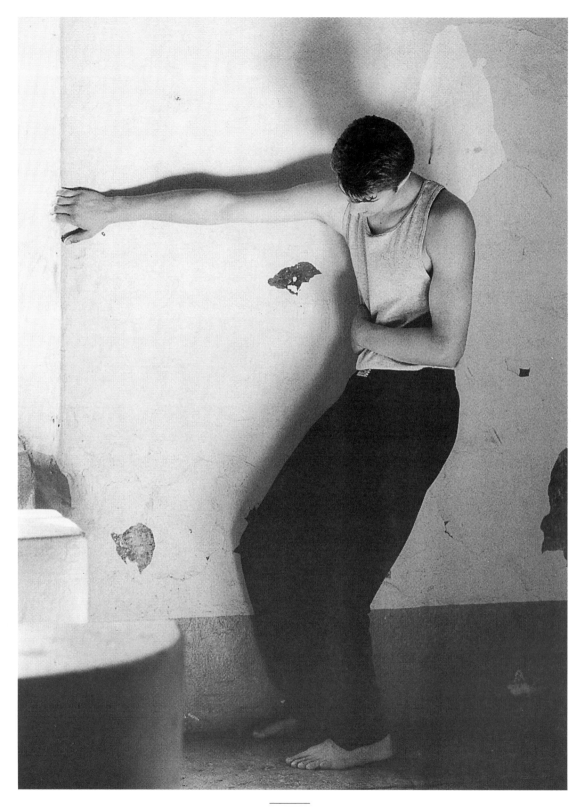

DOORPOST STRETCH

POSITION

Stand straight, beside a door frame at an arm's length from it. Hook your right hand, keeping your arm straight, at shoulder height on to the edge of the door frame. Drop your shoulders and ribs down, drop head slightly left and forward, leading the curve for the spine. Keep the feet parallel.

STEPS

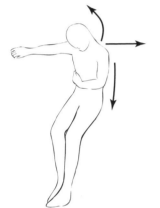

* Focus on the right side of your upper back.

* Breathe into your upper back using Rising-Sun Breathing, and bend the legs.

* As you breathe out, create the stretch by straightening your legs, using the ground point. Tilt your tailbone towards your navel, and keep your head and upper back at the same level.

* Feel the stretch in your upper back. Create a deeper stretch by applying more body weight through the upper back by bending or extending your legs.

NOTE

Visualise your body's flow of movement going toward the floor.

NOTE

You can increase the stretch by placing the right foot in front of you, slightly turned out, while working on the ground point.

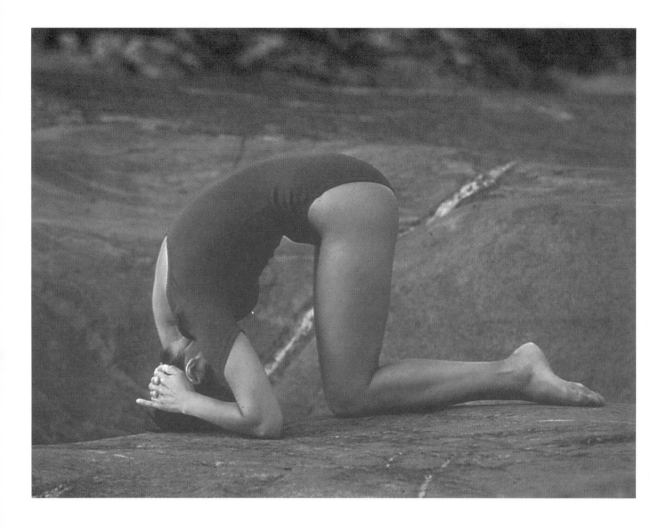

UPSIDE-DOWN STRETCH

POSITION

Kneel and sit back on your heels. Bend your chest down to your knees and put your forehead on the floor in front of you. Clasp your hands behind your head. With your head in place, lift your pelvis so that the legs are straight from the knees at 90 degrees. Be sure not to place your body weight on the head. With the feeling of your head hanging from the neck, use your hands to further tuck the chin into the chest to lengthen the back of the neck. Gently curve your spine upwards. Lift your lower abdominal muscles towards your spine. Turn your tailbone towards your navel. Push the shoulders down.

NOTE

Be sure not to place your body weight on the head but lean against your hands.

STEPS

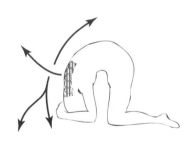

* Focus on your upper back and the back of your neck.

* Use a combination of Half-Moon and Rising-Sun Breathing. Breathe in, directing the pressure of your breathing into the upper back between your shoulderblades.

* As you breathe out, create a gentle stretch by slowly applying more body weight towards the back of your neck, leaning on your hands.

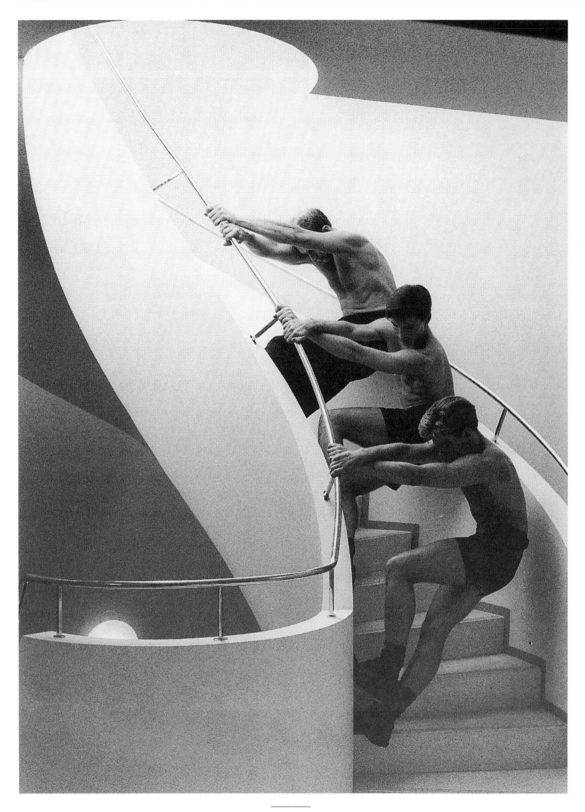

STAIRCASE STRETCH

POSITION

Stand straight facing a staircase or barre, an arm's length from it. Cross your hands right over left on the barre or leave them next to each other. Place your right leg slightly in front of the left. Place it firmly against the wall in front of you. Slightly bend both legs. Turn your right leg out from the hipsocket and turn your tailbone towards your navel. Drop your shoulders and ribs down by pressing down underneath your armpits. Relax your head, tilting it slightly left and forward, following the curve of the spine.

NOTE

By pressing down underneath your armpits you will stabilise your shoulders which is important in order to focus the stretch on the back area.

STEPS

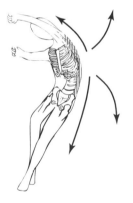

* Focus on the right side of your upper back and all the way down to your lower back.

* Use a combination of Half-Moon and Rising-Sun Breathing, allowing the pressure of the breathing to open your back. While breathing out, engage your abdominal corset.

* Create the stretch by applying body weight towards your back muscles. Slowly bend the right leg, working towards your ground point. As you straighten your leg, tilt your tailbone towards your navel.

NOTE

Find your ground point by visualising your body's flow of movement going towards the floor. Control the stretch with your arms and legs. (However, keep most of the weight on your legs, and the touch of the arms light.) This allows you to apply more body weight gradually through the upper back.

NOTE

Create opposition of movement by rotating your torso towards your right arm.

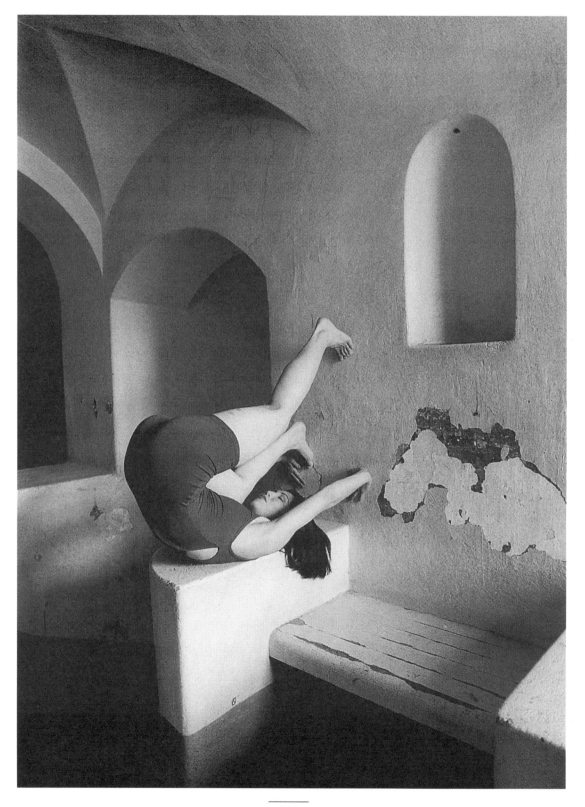

LEG-OVER-HEAD STRETCH

To benefit from this stretch, you need to have enough mobility in your lower back. You can begin from a Standing Lunge (see page 71).

POSITION

Lie on your back with your head at arm's length from a wall. Pull your shoulders down and extend your arms towards the wall, pushing it gently with your hands. Bring your knees to your chest and open them. Breathing out, roll your legs over your head. Initiate this movement from your tailbone. Place your feet on the wall and relax your chest towards the back of your ribs. Extend your right leg up.

STEPS

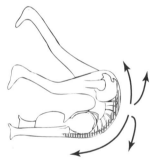

* Focus on your upper back.

* Breathe in, using Half-Moon Breathing.

* As you exhale, engage your abdominal corset. This will drop the weight of your chest down, opening the space between your shoulderblades.

* Create the stretch by gradually pushing against the wall with your hands and feet. Keep lifting your pelvis away from your ribcage by tilting your tailbone towards your navel. Create space between each vertebra as the spine continues curving.

* Stay in the stretch long enough for the sensation of the stretch to travel down toward the lower back area.

NOTE

This stretch may be performed with one leg on the wall at a time. Extend the other leg, rotating it out at the hip, focussing the stretch on either the left or right side of your back.

ARMS

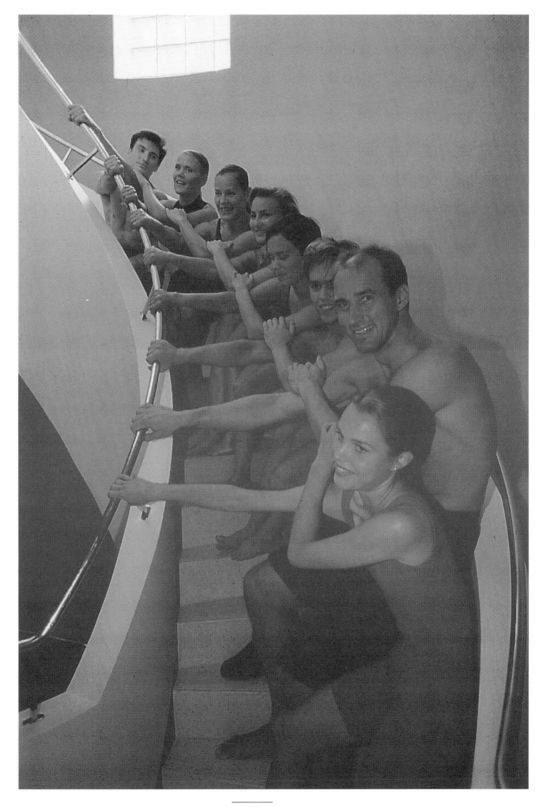

11

BICEPS

1. Biceps Extension
2. Biceps Stretch

MAIN EFFECTS

Shapes your arms, broadens shoulderline, helps the positioning of your shoulders. Frees circulation to your neck, shoulders, arms and hands.

MUSCLE TARGETS

Biceps, Deltoids.

BICEPS EXTENSION

POSITION   Stand beside a wall. Rotate your right arm backwards from the shoulder, dropping your elbow down. Place your palm against the wall at just above shoulder height. Lean on the thumb side of your palm. Step forward on the right leg, transferring your weight on to it. Bend the knee and turn the foot inward. Be sure you maintain your alignment through the centreline. Allow your head to lower, and gradually turn it to the left away from the arm.

NOTE   Stay close to the wall. This allows you to apply enough body weight through your arm while working on your stretch.

NOTE   Keep your shoulder rotated upwards all through the stretch.

STEPS   * Focus on the biceps muscle, located at the front of your arm.

            * Breathe in, using Half-Moon Breathing.

            * While breathing out, create your stretch by rotating your torso away from your arm. Initiate the movement from your tailbone, and readjust your centreline.

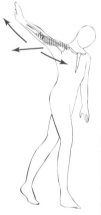

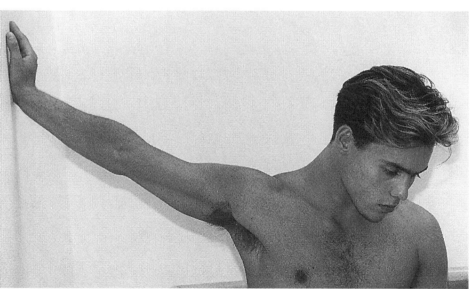

* Turn your legs, starting with the right foot, following with the left. Gradually bend your knees, working with your ground point.

* Continue deepening the stretch, using the breathing, and further rotating the body and legs away from the arm.

N O T E   Since this is a complex muscle in terms of ligament connections, you must use visualisation to find the biceps. Once you can clearly feel the muscle, work slowly to deepen your stretch.

N O T E   Once you have completely turned the body, take the stretch further by deepening the bend in your legs and gradually straighten the arm in this stretched position. Be sure not to lock the elbow, but work your way through the muscle.

BICEPS STRETCH

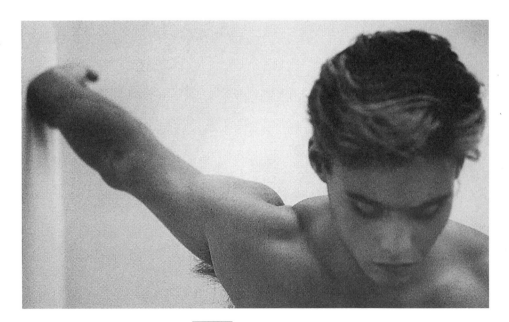

Assume the same position as in Biceps Extension, but place the *back* of your hand against the wall. Work as above.

12

TRICEPS

1. Cross-Body Stretch

2. Triceps Bend

3. Sitting Triceps Extension

MAIN EFFECTS

Shapes your arms, positions
the shoulders, broadens the
shoulderline and opens up the
upper back.

MUSCLE TARGETS

Triceps, Deltoids.

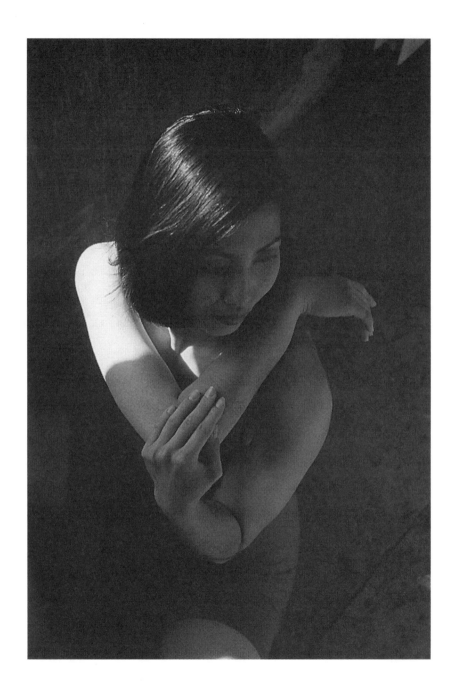

CROSS-BODY STRETCH

POSITION

Sit cross-legged on the floor in an upright position or in a chair with a straight back. Drop your weight on to your sitting bones. Bend the right arm, initiating the movement from the shoulder, and turn the elbow in. Keeping the arm passive, place the palm of the left hand underneath the elbow and then lift the arm across the body towards the left shoulder. Be sure the right arm remains passive. Relax the chest and drop your shoulders.

NOTE

Keeping your back upright is important. If sitting on a chair or sitting against the wall, you can use a pillow against your lower back. If you find it difficult to locate an upright back position, do the stretch standing against the wall with feet parallel.

STEPS

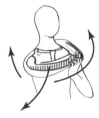

* Focus on the triceps, located at the back of your arms.

* Breathe in, alternating between Half-Moon and Rising-Sun Breathing.

* Create the stretch by gently pressing your right elbow to the left shoulder with your left hand. With the outbreath, create opposition of movement by rotating your torso slightly to the right.

* Deepen the stretch by using your left hand to gently press the right arm closer to the body. Repeat breathing and rotation of the torso.

NOTE

During the stretch keep checking that your right shoulder is down and the right arm is completely passive.

NOTE

This stretch may also be performed focussing on the rhomboids (refer to the section on stretching the upper back).

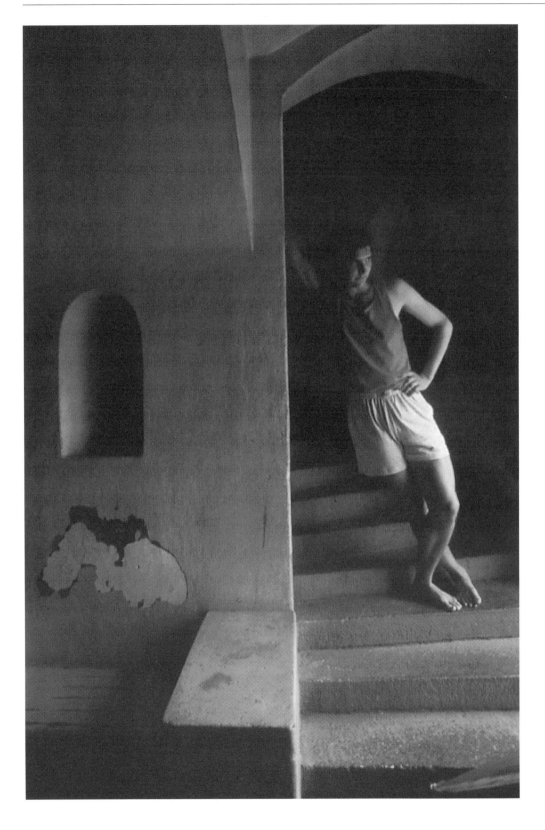

TRICEPS EXTENSION

POSITION   Stand upright with parallel legs in a door frame or next to a wall. Raise the right arm and rotate in from the elbow initiating the movement from your shoulderblade. Drop your hand behind your head, between your shoulderblades. Place the elbow against the wall. Allow the shoulderblade to drop further down against the back. Take your body weight off the left foot by crossing it in front of the right, bending the knee slightly. Gently rest the back of your head against the right arm behind you, keeping the length in your waist. Turn your head slightly to the left and focus your body weight into your right triceps.

NOTE   During the stretch, anchor the shoulderblade down and relax your chest in order to isolate the triceps. Keep your feet close together.

STEPS

* Focus on the triceps.

* Breathe in, alternating between Rising-Sun and Half-Moon Breathing.

* During the outbreath, create the stretch by pulling your right elbow down towards your shoulderblade, keeping the right arm passive.

* Create the stretch by gradually bending the supporting right leg, carefully applying body weight to the triceps.

* As you bend your leg, create opposition of movement by rotating the ribcage away from the arm and inching the head a bit more to the left.

* Breathe out.

NOTE   Continue with this process of breathing and creating opposition of movement. As the stretch deepens imagine the shoulderblade gradually moving down the back and separating from the arm and, thus, lengthening the triceps.

NOTE   Alternate your body weight between both legs to find the position most suitable for you to utilise your body weight.

SITTING TRICEPS EXTENSION

POSITION   Sit cross-legged in a chair with your back upright. Drop your weight on to your sitting-bones. (Refer to positioning in Cross-Body Stretch.) Otherwise follow the positioning and steps as for Triceps Extension.

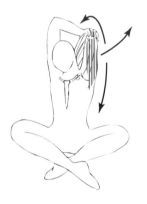

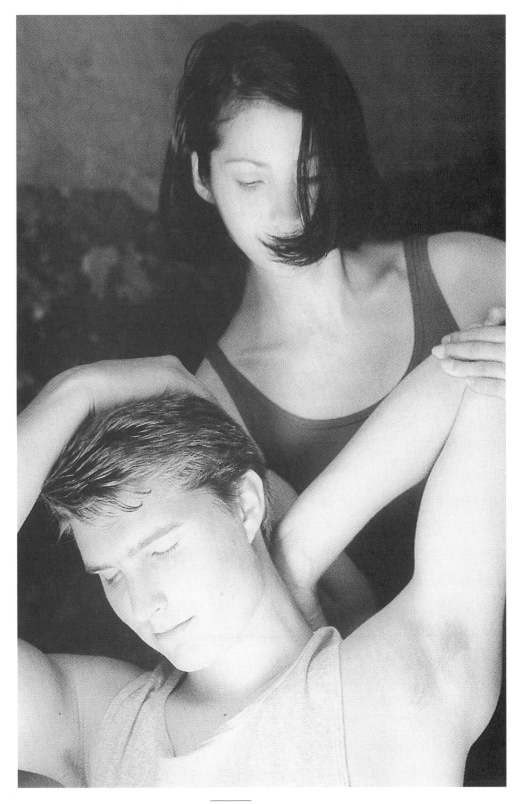

13

LOWER ARM AND HANDS

1. Flexor/Palm Stretch

2. Extensor/Hand Stretch

MAIN EFFECTS

Shapes your arms and wrists, frees circulation through the whole arm area, including the shoulder and neck. Improves flexibility of the hands.

MUSCLE TARGETS

Flexors (humerus, radius, ulna, carpals), Extensors (humerus, radius, ulna, carpals).

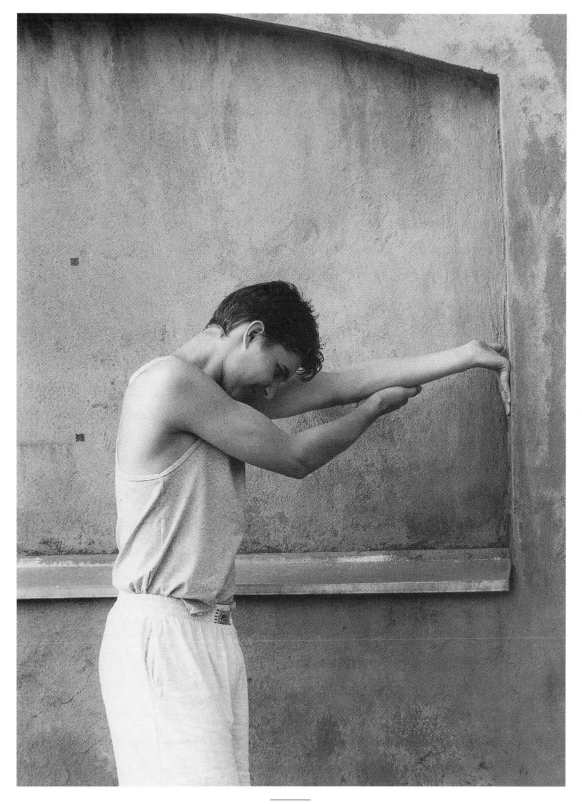

FLEXOR/PALM STRETCH

POSITION

Stand facing a wall. Turn the palm of your left hand upwards, fingers pointing down. Flex your wrist. Extend your arm and place your fingers against the wall.

STEPS

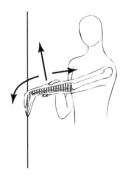

* Focus on the flexors and visualise a line of movement that travels up from the hand to the forearm.

* Breathe normally.

* Relax your hand and fingers. Use the thumb of the right hand to press open the palm and loosen the individual finger bones in the hand.

* Gently lean on to the fingers against the wall, leading them to a more arched position.

* Then move the left hand along the forearm feeling the stretch and the connection with the flexors.

* Deepen the stretch by repeating this sequence of movements, gently increasing the arch of the fingers and palm with each passage.

NOTE

Avoid over-flexing the wrist.

NOTE

With the many nerve endings in the hand, you must manipulate your way through the intense nerve sensations that occur.

EXTENSOR/HAND STRETCH

POSITION   Relax the right hand and extend the arm in front of the body lower than shoulder height, palm and fingers facing downwards. Place the fingers of the left hand on the top of the hand and the thumb on the palm. Pressing the thumb into your palm, use the fingers of your left hand to create opposition of movement.

STEPS
* Focus on the back of the right hand and the muscles between each finger.

* Work on one finger at a time, beginning with the index finger. Create the stretch by pushing the left thumb firmly into the palm of your right hand while slowly bending the top of the hand down. Continue the stretch, eventually bending the finger closer to your wrist.

* After stretching all of your fingers shake the hands out.

14

CHEST

1. Diagonal Press
2. L-Shape Press

MAIN EFFECTS

Opens the chest and shoulderline. Lifts the breasts and tones the underarms. Expands your breathing capacity, increases the circulation to the head, reduces tiredness, neck and shoulder tension and headaches.

MUSCLE TARGETS

Pectoralis Major, Pectoralis Minor.

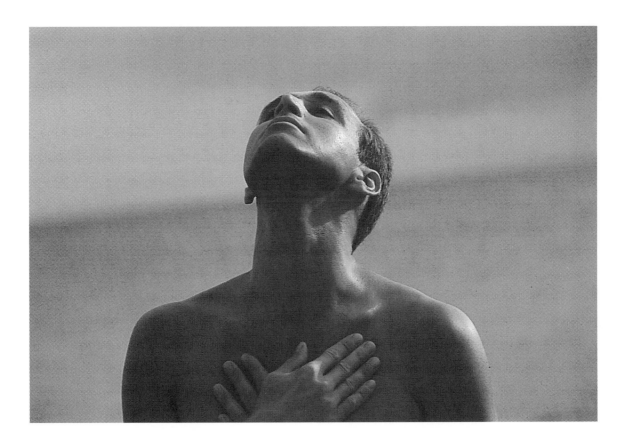

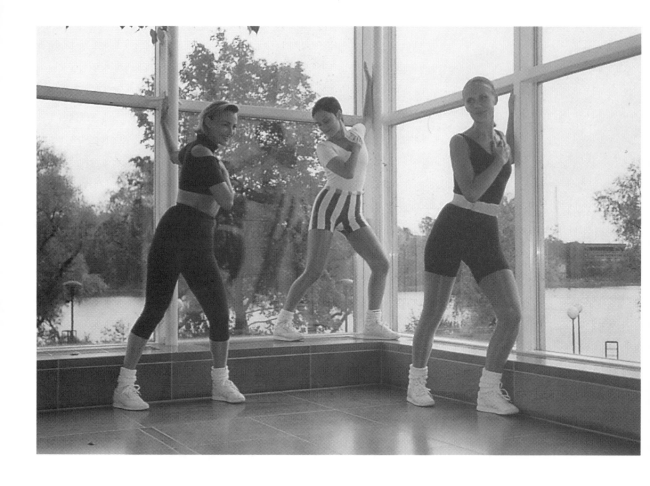

DIAGONAL PRESS

P O S I T I O N   Stand sideways in a doorframe or beside a wall, half an arm's length away. Place your left forearm along the doorframe/wall, elbow bent, fingers up. Lean forward diagonally. Step forward with your left foot, and transfer your weight on to it. Bend your knee slightly. You can place your right hand on your chest to clarify the focus for the stretch.

N O T E   The step forward creates opposition of movement for the stretch.

S T E P S

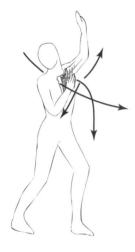

* Focus on the chest and the shoulders.

* Breathe in, using Half-Moon Breathing.

* Create the stretch as you breathe out. Lean forward diagonally and take the muscle to its new length by further bending your legs.

* Now deepen the stretch by rotating your torso and head away from your left arm, initiating the movement from your tailbone. Work with the stretch following the flow of your breathing.

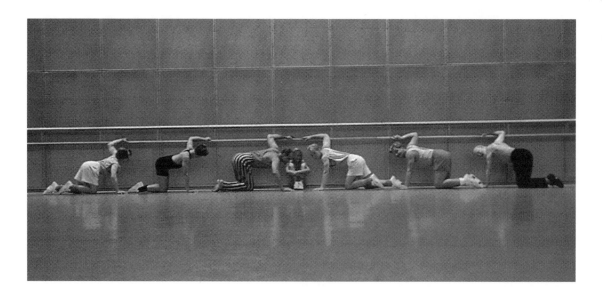

L-SHAPE PRESS

POSITION   Place yourself next to a barre, wall or a table higher than torso level. Begin on your hands and knees, keeping your knees in line with your pelvis at a 90-degree angle. Lift the arm beside the barre diagonally and place it on the barre with the elbow bent. Keep your weight on your supporting arm. Transfer the weight of your back forward.

NOTE   Make sure your elbow is resting slightly higher than and ahead of your chest.

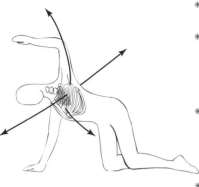

S T E P S

* Focus on the chest.

* Breathe in, using Half-Moon or Rising-Sun Breathing.

* Create the stretch as you breathe out, and lean forward. By bending the supporting arm, you can gradually apply more body weight through the chest.

* Stay with the stretch and deepen it by concentrating on your breathing. With the outbreath, control your centrepoint, engaging your abdominal corset.

* You can further deepen the stretch by extending the inside leg back as you lean forward.

N O T E

As you deepen the stretch, visualise the left shoulderblade moving back to aid in opening up the chest, and drop your head.

V A R I A T I O N

For a more advanced stretch, focus on the deeper layer of chest muscles. You can alternate the positioning of your arm in order to isolate these muscles (for example, extending your arm forward).

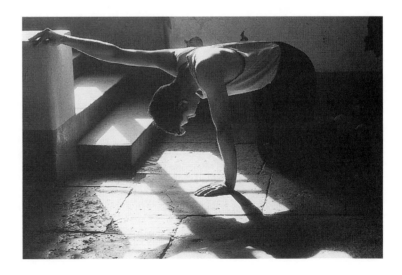

15

NECK AND FACE

1. Long-Neck Stretch

2. Side-to-Side Neck/Face Stretch

3. Cross-Arm Neck Stretch

4. Curved-Neck Stretch

5. Jaw Stretch

MAIN EFFECTS

Increases blood circulation to the head and face, lifts the face and neck, releasing tension in the neck, shoulder and upper back area. Improves posture.

MUSCLE TARGETS

Platysma, Upper Trapezius, Sternocleidomastoid, Myohyoid.

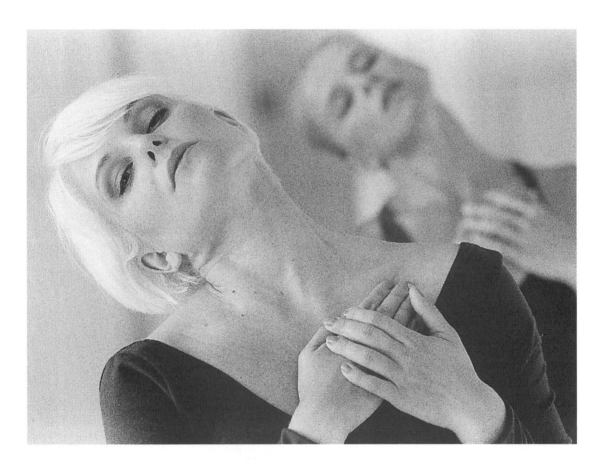

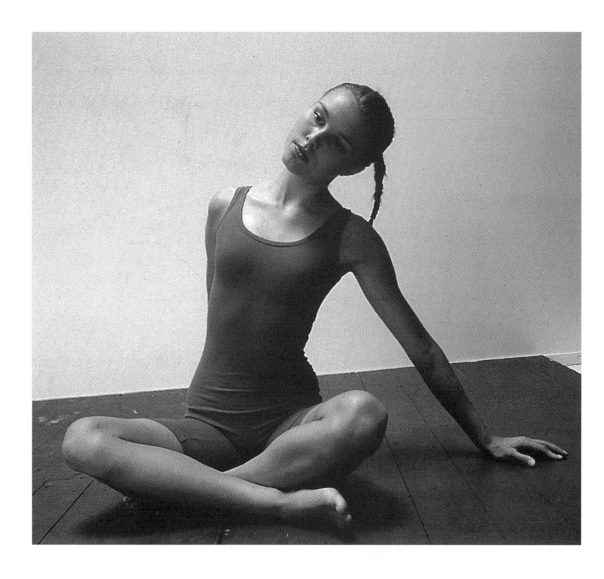

LONG-NECK STRETCH

POSITION

Sit upright in a cross-legged position, or on a chair. Rotate your shoulders back and lift your chest upwards. Extend your left arm to the side, placing your hand on the floor. Tilt your head to the left, while lifting your cheek towards the ceiling. Relax your right arm.

STEPS

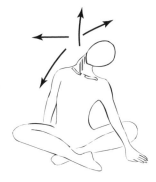

* Focus on the right side of your neck.

* Breathe in, using Rising-Sun Breathing.

* Create the stretch and opposition of movement by reaching your right arm in a diagonal slightly behind your shoulder. Further relax your head to the left.

* Breathe out, emptying the upper part of your lungs. Keep your head in this relaxed position and deepen the stretch by slowly extending and lowering your right arm in slight movements.

NOTE

Allowing your head to lead the curve of the torso to the left will also add to the depth of your stretch. Continue rotating your shoulder back.

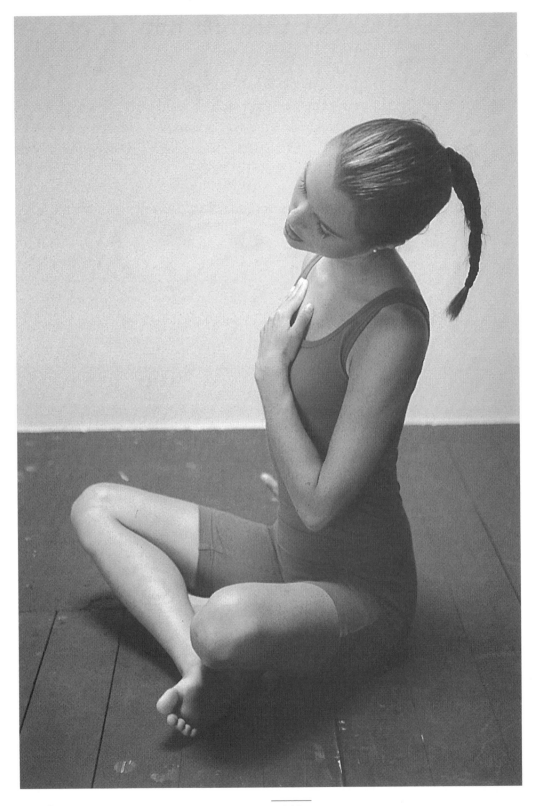

SIDE-TO-SIDE NECK/FACE STRETCH

POSITION

Sit cross-legged on the floor with a straight back. Tilt your head to the left, lifting your cheek to the ceiling. Rotate your shoulders back and lift your chest upward. Place your left hand on your right collarbone and gently pull down the muscles around it.

NOTE

Using your left hand to gently pull on the collarbone area helps to emphasise opening the right side of your neck.

STEPS

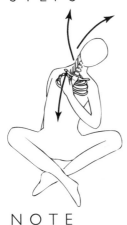

* Focus on the neck muscles running along the right side of your jawline down to your collarbone.

* Breathe in, using Rising-Sun Breathing.

* Create the stretch by relaxing your head and using your hands to gently pull and separate your head from your collarbone. Feel the opening of the side of your neck.

* As you breathe out, deepen the stretch further by lifting your right cheek further upwards.

NOTE

If you would like to progress the stretch, gently lower your left arm to the floor and behind your body. You may also use both hands on the muscles of the right collarbone area to deepen the stretch.

CROSS-ARM NECK STRETCH

POSITION

Sit cross-legged on the floor or on a chair. Keep your back upright (see Note). Extend both arms down, palms up, rotate your elbows towards each other and cross right over the left. Lift your right arm with your left, underneath the elbow, keeping your elbows crossed. Place your left hand on your right wrist, palms facing each other. Tilt your head to the left. Be sure your right arm remains passive. Relax your ribcage and shoulders

NOTE

The upright positioning of your back is important. If sitting on a chair or sitting against the wall, you can use a pillow against your lower back. If you find it difficult to locate a straight back position, do the stretch standing against the wall with feet parallel.

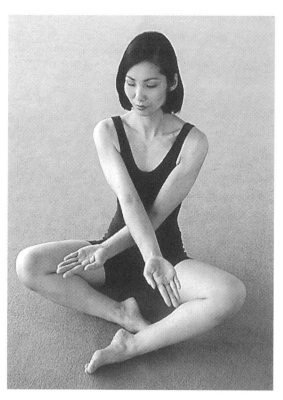
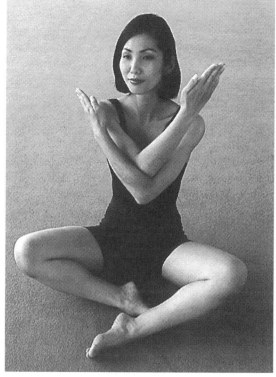

STEPS

* Focus on the muscles either at the side or back of your neck towards your shoulderblade area.

* Breathe in, alternating between Half-Moon and Rising-Sun Breathing, and focus your breath on your upper back.

* Breathe out and create the stretch by actively using your left hand to press your right arm down towards the floor. Relax your chest and drop your shoulders further down.

* Continue deepening the stretch by keeping your right arm passive as you slowly lift it up and down with the left arm. During the DELAY of your outbreath, gently press your right arm further down with your left hand.

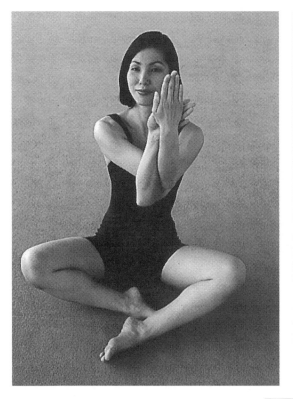
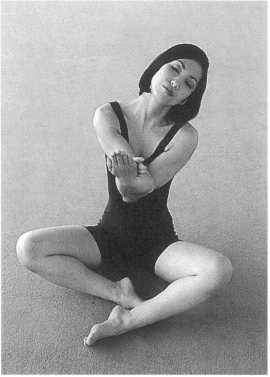

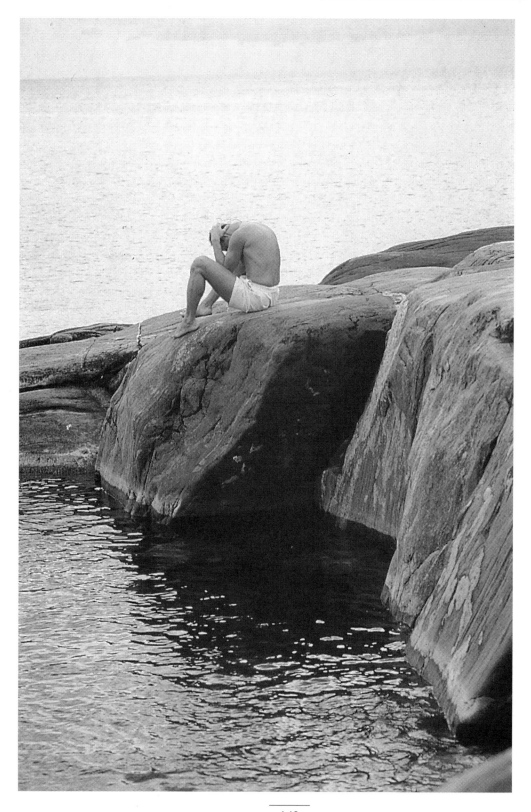

CURVED-NECK STRETCH

POSITION

Sit cross-legged and upright (see Note on positioning of Cross-Arm Neck Stretch), and focus forward. Create length in the back of your neck by tilting your chin down. Interlock your fingers and place both hands behind your head at a level above your ears. Bring your elbows together. Allow your neck, arms and upper back to be passive.

STEPS

* Focus on the back of your neck.

* Use Rising-Sun Breathing. Focus your breath between the shoulderblades.

* Create your stretch as you breathe out, using the weight of your arms to bring your chin closer to your chest. This will increase the curve of your upper back.

* Try to fully empty the upper part of your lungs, engaging your abdominal corset. This also creates opposition of movement. Allow the pressure of the next inhalation to deepen your stretch.

* Work on the stretch for a good length of time (a minimum of 3 minutes).

NOTE

If this stretch feels as though it is creating too much pressure, you may ease it up at various intervals while you work towards a deeper stretch.

NOTE

Vary the position of the head to the right and left diagonals.

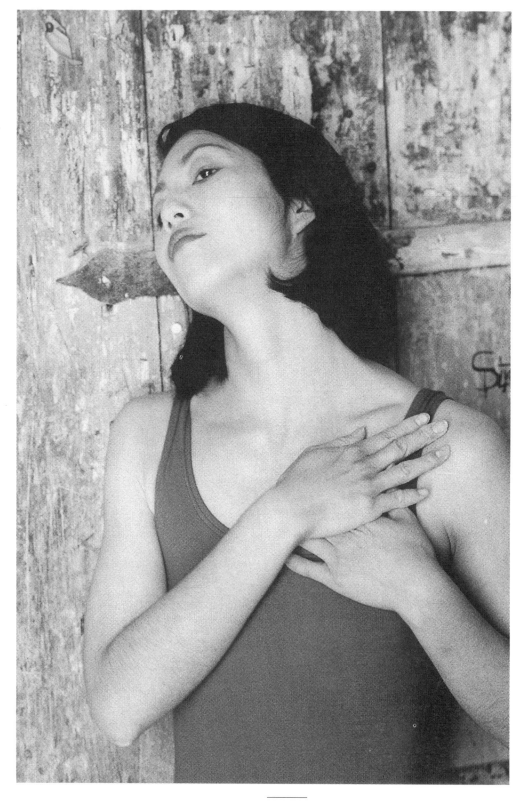

JAW STRETCH

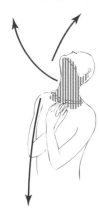

POSITION

Stand or sit cross-legged. Roll your shoulders back and drop them down. Lift your chest. Lengthen the front of your neck by slightly lifting your chin upward (do not close off the back of your neck). Place both your hands at the centre of your collarbone area, one on top of the other.

STEPS

* Focus on the neck muscles running from the top of your chest to your lower jaw line.

* Breathe in, using Rising-Sun Breathing. As you breathe in, create the stretch and opposition of movement by using your hands at your collarbone area to pull your neck muscles down. To feel them sliding over your collarbone, further lift your chin.

* As you exhale, increase opposition of movement to deepen the stretch. To feel the stretch at the top of your throat, swallow.

* Continue focussing on the side of your jaw by turning your head slightly.

NOTE

By swallowing you may become aware of the amount of tension you carry in the throat area underneath your chin. This stretch is suitable for addressing the tightness of the upper throat that results in a double chin.

PARTNERWORK

Working with another person helps you to stretch your muscles further in a more concentrated way. The element of touch can be used to help focus, relax, and elongate the chosen muscle. In partnerwork, touch is used with the five elements to reach the desired stretch.

To achieve this there must be trust, cooperation and an open line of communication between the two of you, whether you are the assistant or the recipient. This is both you and your partner's responsibility. If you are the person assisting a stretch, be clear about your focus and the target. The process of working as an assistant can contribute to your sensitivity and understanding of the exercises. If you are the person being stretched, bear in mind that only you know the sensations of your body. Use the element of touch as a positive addition to stretching. It not only deepens each stretch, but it can also act as a source of comfort, relaxation and enjoying one another's company.

You can observe from the following photographs that, once you master the fundamentals of deep stretching, you can then create variations on the stretches which will be suitable for your own body, and which will allow you to explore and enjoy the whole concept of stretching.

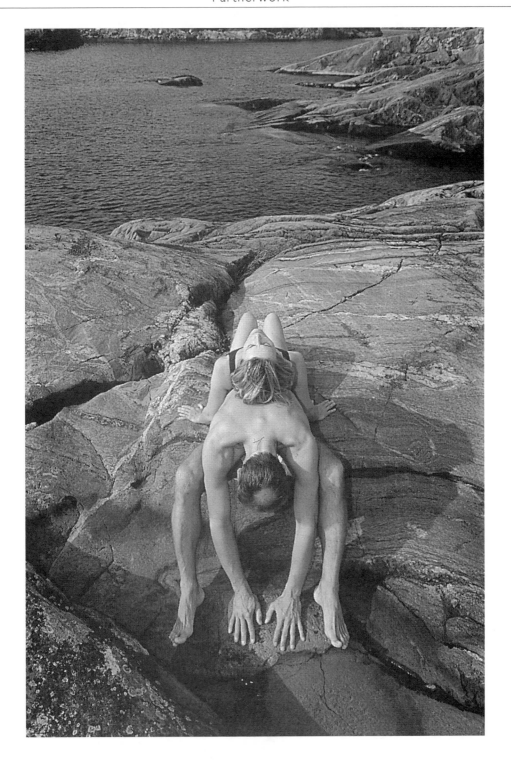

HOW TO TOUCH

Touch is an instant form of communication. When using it in deep stretching it must be firm, reliable and sensitive at the same time. There are two principles to follow when assisting by touch. First, touch is always applied going from light to heavy. Second, it is applied as a sustained and controlled movement, not a sudden one.

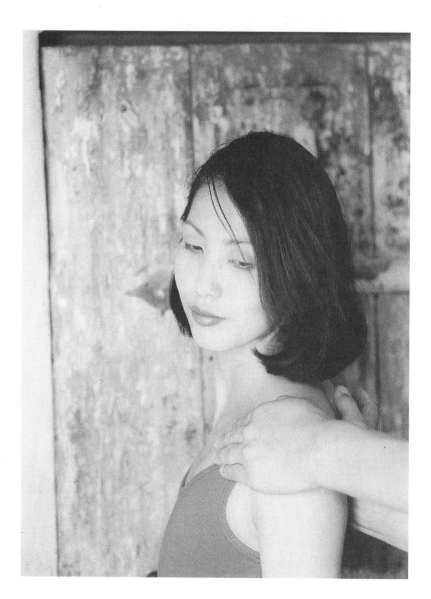

1. FOCUS TOUCH

This can be used to pinpoint precisely the area being worked on or to assist with breathing. This is a practical way of helping you connect with your blind spots.

The assistant gently places the whole of their hand and fingers, or both hands, on the area of focus, whichever is appropriate for the exercise.

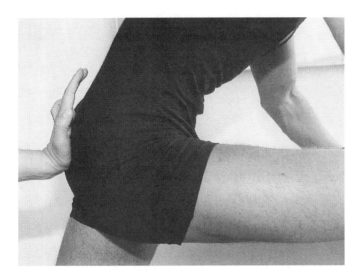

2. PRESSURE TOUCH

In this, the assistant applies weight to deepen a stretch or help with breathing. It is helpful for relaxing pelvis, hamstring and shoulderline muscles into a new length.

The assistant must be clear about the focus of the stretch. He/she places their hands on the muscle or muscles to apply body weight and deepen the stretch. Then additional weight is applied at the DELAY moments between breaths when the muscle releases its biting point.

3. SUPPORT TOUCH

The assistant provides support or resistance for either stretching or breathing. He/she places their hands or body in a position that acts as a support platform to lean on. This allows you and the muscle to relax into the stretch. The assistant should apply enough resistance for you to work against, but not so much that it inhibits the movement of the stretch. This is useful for waistline and pelvic stretches.

BREATHING

RISING-SUN BREATHING

ASSISTANT Use Focus Touch, placing a hand on your partner's chest. Allow him or her to breathe in. As he/she breathes out, use a gentle Pressure Touch to help him/her to empty the upper part of the lungs fully.

RECIPIENT Use your partner's touch to focus on fully filling or emptying your upper lung.

HALF-MOON BREATHING

ASSISTANT Sit behind your partner. Use Support Touch, placing your hands around the lower part of your partner's ribs. Create a slight resistance as he/she breathes into the lower part of their lungs. Apply Pressure Touch as he/she breathes out, engaging the abdominal corset to empty the deeper part of the lungs fully.

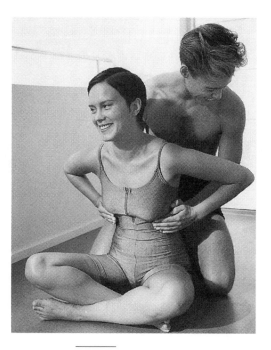

LEGS

L - P U L L

ASSISTANT   Stand behind your partner who is stretching his/her right hamstring. Use Support and Pressure Touches. Place your right hand for a support on the back top of your partner's hamstring. Place your left hand for a Pressure Touch on the lower left side of your partner's back. Elongate your partner's hamstring by creating opposition of movement with the placement of your hands. Using your ground point, apply body weight through your left hand forward, and pull your right hand toward you simultaneously.

NOTE   As the assistant, your target is to increase the length of the hamstrings located from the back of the knee to the sitting bones.

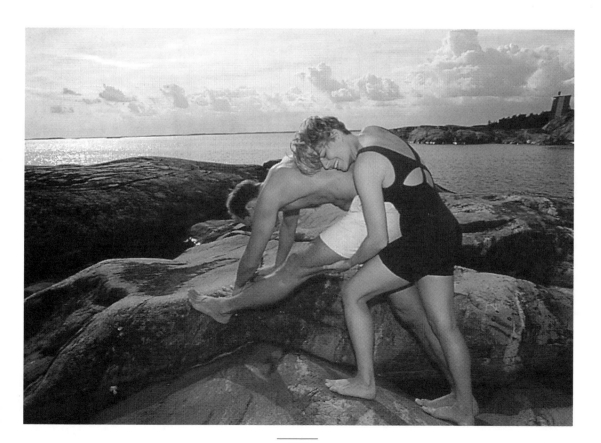

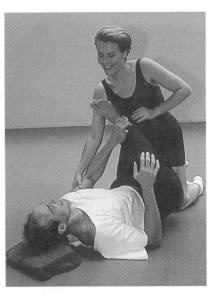

PELVIS & BUTTOCKS
SITTING LUNGE –
Variation

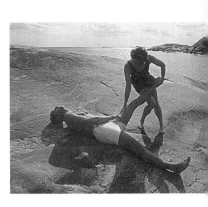

LEGS
INNER THIGHS –
LYING V Variation

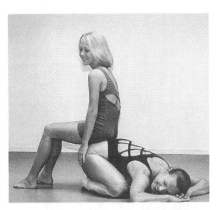

BACK
LOWER BACK STRETCH

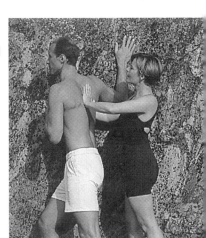

CHEST
DIAGONAL PRESS

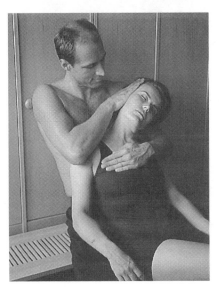

NECK & FACE
SIDE-TO-SIDE
NECK STRETCH

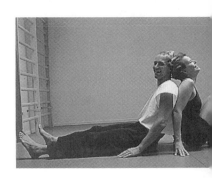

CENTRING COOL DOWN

At the end of each stretching session always re-centre and calm yourself.

1. Re-establish your centreline. Lie down on your back and rock on your pelvis by tilting it backwards and forwards five times (see Warming Up).

2. Take one each of a Balloon, Rising-Sun and Half-Moon breath.

3. Extend your arms and legs, and reach them away from your spine. Press the back of your ribs into the floor. Breathe in using Half-Moon Breathing. Breathe out, engaging your abdominal corset. Hold your breath to a count of three. Relax and repeat three times.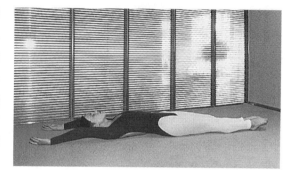

4. Place your fingertips on your forehead. Give yourself a gentle massage around your eyes.

5. Consciously relax the muscles behind and around your eyes. Open your mouth wide as if yawning and open your eyes as wide as possible. Close your mouth and eyes tightly, then repeat. Relax your face.

6. Breathe in and out naturally. Use your mind to travel through your body as you relax your pelvis, your legs, your back and upper back, abdominals, arms, chest, neck and back to your face.

7. Imagine all your tensions and worries flowing out of your body on to the floor. Just listen to your breathing.

8. Take with you only your strength and energy.

9. For the moment be satisfied with your work.

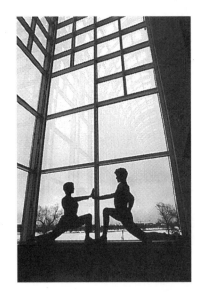

Thank you for your time...

MARJA PUTKISTO